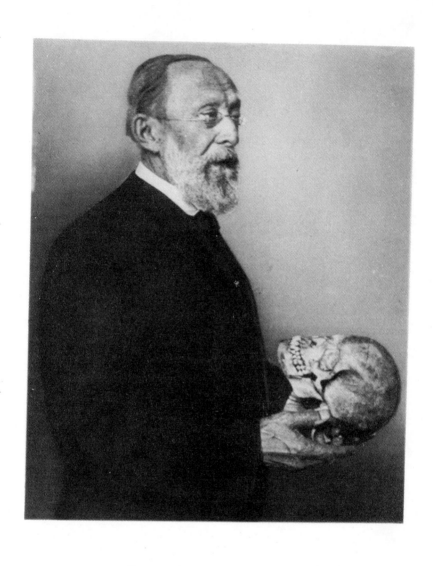

Rudolf Virchow (1821-1902)
Reproduced from Virchow's *Archiv* through the courtesy of
Prof. Otto Lubarsch

A HISTORY OF
PATHOLOGY

BY

ESMOND R. LONG, Ph.D., M.D.

Emeritus Professor of Pathology
Henry Phipps Institute
University of Pennsylvania

Formerly Professor of Pathology
University of Chicago

DOVER PUBLICATIONS, INC., NEW YORK

Published in Canada by General Publishing Company, Ltd., 30 Lesmill Road, Don Mills, Toronto, Ontario.

Published in the United Kingdom by Constable and Company Limited, 10 Orange Street, London W. C. 2.

This Dover edition, first published in 1965, is an enlarged and corrected republication of the work first published by the Williams & Wilkins Company in 1928. The author has prepared a new Preface and an Appendix (Recent Trends in Pathology, 1929-1963) especially for this Dover edition.

Library of Congress Catalog Card Number: 64-15513

Manufactured in the United States of America

Dover Publications, Inc.
180 Varick Street
New York, N. Y. 10014

Foreword to the First Edition

As good wine needs no bush, so it is always an act of supererogation to devise a foreword to a worthwhile book, unless by a foreign author. The only reasons which can be assigned for running counter to settled conviction in this case are, that here is the first definite and systematic account of the subject in English and that our author has succeeded in the execution of his plan through his competence, his praiseworthy industry and a spirit ever ready to correct errors pointed out or ascertained. Dr. Long, a pupil of Wells and Hektoen and Professor of Pathology in the University of Chicago, has written this volume for the benefit of his classes. He is entirely right in his conviction that "nothing gives a better perspective of the subject than an appreciation of the steps by which it has reached its present state." That the space-time purview is the best check upon the bewildering masses of detail, now presented to students in all branches of medicine, has become settled conviction since Osler first essayed this method in the hospital wards. There is hardly any good medical teacher to-day who does not supplement the detailed presentation of his subject by its historic milestones and landmarks, its triumphs and failures, its pathways and pitfalls. For teaching of this practical kind, the earlier sketches of such masters as Virchow (1895) or Chiari (1903) are hardly adequate, and Edgar Goldschmid's History of Pathological Illustration (Leipzig, 1925), while in the newer trend of visualization, is essentially an album of reference, consciously patterned after Choulant.

Dr. Long has arranged this survey in twelve compact chapters, illustrating the different new departures in the progress of pathology. Like so many other branches of medicine, the subject had no continuous evolution but progressed by fits and starts, the moments of energy (or inertia) being variously the humoral doctrine of antiquity, the coming of the judicial post-mortem in the Middle Ages, the invention of printing, the rise of modern anatomy (Leonardo and Vesalius), the evolution of anatomical illustration from pen drawing and woodcut to steel-plate and photograph, the systematizing tendencies of the 18th century, the correlation of clinical data with post-mortem findings (Morgagni), experimentation (John Hunter, Magendie), the beginnings of histology (Bichat, Henle), microscopy, the cell-theory (Schwann, Virchow), the rise of neurology (Charcot), of bacteriology (Pasteur, Koch), of serology and immunology (Metchnikoff, Ehrlich), of endocrinology (Brown-Séquard) and of biochemistry (Emil Fischer). Apart from the greater masters, the names which shine out as "values" in this story—Benivieni, Fernel, Plater, Coiter, Dodoens, Schenck von Grafenberg, Severino, Tulp, Pieter Pauw, Wepfer, Bonet, Kerkring, Blankaart, Vieussens, Senac, Sandifort, Gaub, Baillie, Bayle, Lobstein, Cruveilhier, Rayer, Carswell, Horner, Vetter, Weichselbaum, Paltauf, Chiari, Recklinghausen, Villemin, Stricker, Weigert, Ziegler, Zenker, Paget, Delafield, Prudden—are essentially different from the routine landmarks in a straight history of general medicine, and illustrate Sudhoff's view that the history of a special discipline can be properly written by an expert only. In consequence of the rise of bacteriology (about 1875-1900), gross and microscopic (descriptive) pathology were thrown into the background and ceased to be influential for nearly half a century. The antagonism of Virchow and his school to Koch was not personal but concerned with anticipation of this tendency. The bitter hostility of Recklinghausen toward Naunyn at Strassburg would probably have been mitigated had Naunyn been a Virchow pupil. During the World War, it was hard to find medical officers who could perform a post-mortem section on occasion. The remarkable organizing abilities displayed by Aschoff during the war period have given a fresh impetus to pathology. In this newer dispensation, the morphological (descriptive), biochemical and experimental phases, in other words, form, substance and force, are coming to be recognized as interdependent and correlated, as in physics or chemistry. "The physician, who recognizes the imperative duty of dwelling in things, ought to guard himself from being supposed to mean only things that stand still; his sphere is, on the contrary, with things in motion—he is a master of dynamics" (Allbutt).

To go into the remoter origins of pathology, to inquire whence, why and how it came into being, is to go back to the most fundamental questionings of the human mind. Osler has said that "the quest for righteousness is Oriental, the quest for knowledge Occidental." After Gautama had his first sight of a decrepit old man, a loathsome disease, a putrid corpse, he rode out into the moonlight to seek the pathway of renunciation as well as of enlightenment. His solution of the great problem, "What is the cause of pain and sorrow, disease and death?", was the foundation of one of the greater religions of the world. The same dark problem was considered, it is true, by Æschylus and Sophocles, and with similar ethical reactions, but Hippocrates by the bedside, Galen staring at the robber's skeleton, took a far different line from the noble Rajput prince. For the question raised by Sakya Muni, in his mournful vigils under the Bo tree, is the very pulse and *raison d'être* of pathology, the science of suffering and disease. The probable (or presumable) reactions of primitive man have been traced with skill and intelligence by Sudhoff. The misery of the sick patient suggested a demon inside his body, but it was noticeable that flowing blood is usually associated with violent death or with the discomfort of menstruation, with epistaxis, with internal troubles (bloody urine and faeces) and above all with wounds. "Blood flows from wounds, as also from the nose, the eyelids, the mouth, the vessels, the sexual and excretory orifices . . . blood is in fact everywhere." The same reasoning, applied to tears, sputum, cerumen, urine, faeces, semen, the menses, vomitus, pus and mucus, led inevitably to humoralism, already crystallized in the *sualu* or "mucus-series" of diseases in the Assyro-Babylonian medical texts (Küchler). From Greece came the number-lore of Pythagoras, his theory that the universe is made up of opposing elements, and the successive views of the Ionian philosophers, viz., that water, earth, air and fire are the primordial elements of being. In the poetic fragments of Empedocles,[1] these elements are presently combined with their outstanding physical qualities (wet, dry, cold, warm) into an archaic physical chemistry and physiology:

> And first the fourfold root of all things hear:
> .... For knowledge gained
> Makes strong the soul. For as before I spake,
> Naming the utter goal of these my words,
> I will report a twofold truth. Now grows
> The One from many into being, now

1 Translated by Professor William Ellery Leonard, Chicago, 1908.

Even from the One disparting come the Many,—
Fire, Water, Earth and awful heights of Air.

. . . .

For from these elements hath budded all
That was or is or evermore shall be.
All trees and men and women, beasts and birds,
And fishes nourished in deep waters, aye,
The long-lived gods, in honors excellent.

. . . .

First rose mere lumps of earth with rude impress,
That had their share of Water and of Warm.
These then by Fire (in upward zeal to reach
Its kindred Fire in heaven) were shot aloft,
Albeit not yet had they revealed a form
Of lovely limbs, nor yet a human cry,
Nor secret member, common to the male.

. . . .

Into clean wombs the seeds are poured, and when
Therein they meet with Cold, the birth is girls;
And boys, when contrariwise they meet with Warm.

. . . .

On the tenth day, in month the eighth, the blood
Becomes white pus.

From cold, dry earth, cold, wet water, hot, dry fire and warm, moist air it was, in fact, but a step to sundry body-fluids noted by the Babylonians, viz., hot, moist blood, cold, moist phlegm, hot dry (yellow) bile and cold, dry (black) bile. From these permutations and combinations came the humoral pathology, which influenced European medical practice even into the seventeenth century, as evidenced by countless passages in the Elizabethan, Jacobean and Caroline dramatists alone.

Although intended primarily for students, this book can be cordially recommended to any physician who wishes to know the origins and evolution of the basic discipline of scientific medicine. The scheme of illustration alone is highly instructive, indicating the enormous amount of devoted, self-sacrificing labor which has helped to make our profession the competent body of scientific men it is today.

F. H. GARRISON

Army Medical Museum
August 9, 1928

Preface to the Dover Edition

A History of Pathology was first published by the Williams and
Wilkins Company of Baltimore in 1928. The author recalls with
pleasure his cordial relations with the officers of that publishing
house and wishes to express his appreciation of the generous en-
dorsement they have given, in courteous correspondence with Mr.
Hayward Cirker, President of Dover Publications, Inc., to publication of the book in soft covers. Mr. Cirker's championship of
books in paperback binding has set a new style and intrigued the
interest not only of the reading public but also of publishers of
books in the older traditional format.

It is hoped by the author that this paperback edition of *A
History of Pathology* will increase its availability for medical
students, who are meeting heavily increased expenses for text-
books in the midst of rising costs for medical education in general. It is perhaps not too much to hope that the volume in its
new form will have some appeal for their teachers also, as a
medium for picturing with desired brevity the background of
their science. The need for background information is no less
now than it was a generation ago. In fact it is probably greater.
In a plethora of technical detail, the historical record is a stabiliz-
ing element, providing useful perspective for a course that has
been successful in the past.

The changes that have been made in the present edition are
relatively simple. The major element has been the addition of an
Appendix in which the principal achievements of the last third of
a century are set forth briefly, and important trends in progress
emphasized. This has been attempted more by pertinent illustration than by chronicle in detail. Coupled with this is some
indication, in the light of events outlined in the old edition, of
advances now being made by pathology, and some prediction of
the course it may be expected to follow in the future.

Otherwise, modifications have been small. Where interim research has cleared up uncertainties or added significant new

facts, appropriate changes have been made in the text. In the original edition events were recorded in a spirit of youthful enthusiasm and, admittedly, with hyperbole in expression. Hero-worship was commoner a generation ago than in these days of harder realism. This tone has been allowed to stand, for the events of the story, in whatever way they are described, are inspiring.

Few will take issue with Colonel Fielding H. Garrison's designation, in his Foreword to the first edition, of pathology as the basic discipline of scientific medicine. It is not surprising that in the course of recent years pathology has greatly broadened its scope and amalgamated on an increasing scale with other fundamental disciplines of medicine. It would have been surprising, and lamentable too, if it had not done so.

E. R. L.

University of Pennsylvania
Philadelphia, Penna., July 31, 1964

Preface to the First Edition

This book is intended primarily for the medical student. In a day of increasingly crowded medical curriculum the details the student is expected to master must inevitably confuse him, unless he has some comprehensive outlook for his facts. A few years of teaching pathology have led to the conviction that nothing gives a better perspective of the subject than an appreciation of the steps by which it has reached its present state.

Moreover an honest presentation of pathology compels the constant admission of uncertainty with regard to its details, which may lose the student's confidence, unless he is made to understand that the whole development of the science has been but a conquest of similar uncertainties. It may surprise him that the greatest masters in the subject have made some of the worst mistakes, but on second thought there is much encouragement in the revelation.

Of necessity an historical account must be largely biographical. Men and their books have built pathology. Yet without a point of view which takes account of the major social movements of general history, no real conception of the historical development of any subject is possible. Unfortunately a small book of this character, already compressed to the exclusion of much interesting and informing detail on its own subject matter, cannot hope to take much account of general history, and must leave that to other sources.

The biographical approach almost inevitably opens the way to errors in the proper assignment of credit for discoveries. Undoubtedly such are present in this book. The chief effort has been made to give credit to those men and schools whose discoveries were influential, even though that success may have been merely the good fortune of a ripe time. Because of the difficulty of evaluating the achievements of our own time, recent discoveries have for the most part been omitted.

In the preparation of this small volume I have received help from many quarters. The staff of the John Crerar Library have been particularly kind in giving me easy access to their rich material and temporary possession of rare volumes for reproduction of the cuts. Professors Singer, Lubarsch and Loewenstein have sent me material from abroad for inclusion among the figures. Professor Hektoen has made valuable suggestions with regard to the illustrations and loaned me useful material. Other colleagues and friends have aided with the manuscript, corrected errors and made valuable suggestions.

I have drawn freely on the many excellent publications in the field of medical history, too many, I fear, for individual acknowledgment. I am particularly indebted to the chapter on the History of Pathology by Hanns Chiari in Puschmann's *Handbook of the History of Medicine,* to Professor Neuburger's *History of Medicine* and above all to Lt. Col. Fielding H. Garrison's *Introduction to the History of Medicine,* which has been of value in every chapter in this book. Colonel Garrison has also taken a personal interest in improving the text, which has been extremely helpful. For all of this aid I wish to express my thanks.

E. R. L.

The University of Chicago
Chicago, Ill., June 1, 1928

Contents

Illustrations

TEXT FIGURES

PLATES

CHAPTER I

The Pathology of Antiquity

Pathology has always been only the attempt to understand the nature of those deviations from normal health which we call disease. The first pathologist was the first man to reason with uncommon care upon the physical ailments afflicting him as he emerged from the condition of the brutes. As men became gregarious the natural division of labor among groups led to the separation of a profession who made a special inquiry into the causes, as well as the best mode of treatment, of illness. We meet these specialists at the opening of historical times, and see them in their early state in the primitive peoples of today.

Archaeological discoveries of recent years have furnished a rich record of the observations of prehistoric peoples on the gross features of external disease. In antiquity the healing art was intimately bound with theological practice. The sick visited the temples of the gods for relief from their ills and pains. If convalescence, real or fancied, followed their prayers, tokens of acknowledgment of the divine aid in the form of small sculptured or molded human shapes portraying the diseased parts, were frequently left in the temple collections. Very good marble and terra cotta representations of hernias, tumors of the female breast, abdominal dropsy, obesity, varicose veins, ulcers and swellings of the skin, and other external lesions, were thus preserved, testifying to the anatomical knowledge and point of view of these remote times.

In ancient Egypt medical science was dominated by two classes of educated men, medical priests trained in the contents of the Hermetic books and physician specialists. The priest was the superior of the two, and medical thought grew up with him. Explanations of disease took on a theistic and demonistic tinge, and the driving out of devils, so familiar in the writings of the much-captured Hebrews, who drew many of their intellectual concepts from their frequent masters, the Egyptians, was one of the most important procedures in the early priestly practice of medicine in Egypt.

Yet even in the old papyri on the magic arts some objective analysis of disease can be discerned. One of these ancient records refers to a specific demon of sickness as a "brother of blood, companion of pus and father of malignant swelling." Thus early do we see attention called to certain of the elements of inflammation, which from earliest times and in every period has ranked as the leading problem of pathology.

Moreover, with the obvious selective localization of disease constantly before their eyes, as in ophthalmia, dysentery and various skin diseases, it was inevitable that human ailment should be correlated with anatomy of a sort. The earlier Egyptians apparently felt freer to develop the anatomical side of medical science than did their successors of the later dynasties. As early as 4000 B.C., before the building of the pyramids, Atho-this, son and successor of Menes, founder of the first dynasty, as we are told by the historian Manetho, wrote books on medicine, the first of which treated of anatomy. Long before the time from which written records survive, a conventional anatomy curiously symmetrical in its exposition of the human frame, and inaccurate to a degree precluding much practical use as far as internal parts were concerned, was available to the Egyptian medical student and priest.

The vascular system received the most attention and its abnormalities were not neglected. What we now call aneurysms were noted and comments made on them, and attention was called in medical writings to the accumulation of blood in inflamed parts. The method of anatomical systematization, beginning with the head and its disorders and proceeding methodically downward, is, however, the one enduring contribution of Egyptian anatomical science.

The most important sources for information on Egyptian medicine are the Papyrus Ebers (about 1550 B.C.), deciphered by the German Egyptologist Georg Ebers, and the still more ancient Edwin Smith Papyrus, a surgical treatise with case records from the seventeenth century B.C., translated by Breasted. From these we learn of bone injuries, traumatic and spontaneous, of eye disease like the trachoma which still scourges the Nile Valley, of ulcerating lumps that might be construed as cancer, of fatty tumors, of intestinal parasites and dysentery, of hookworm, of amputation, lithotomy, bandaging, cupping, venesection, cir-

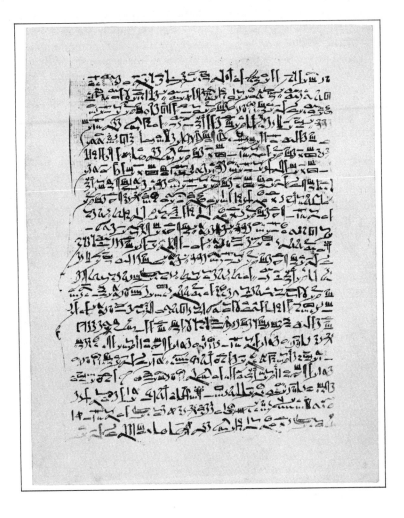

A PORTION OF THE EDWIN SMITH PAPYRUS DEALING WITH
INJURIES OF THE HEAD
Through the courtesy of Prof. James Breasted

cumcision, and castration, and a stupendous drug therapy which
gave us our very word "chemistry," the magic science of Chemi,
or ancient Egypt, the Black land.

Nevertheless the sixteen-foot roll forming the Edwin Smith

Papyrus, and the one hundred and ten hieroglyphed columns of the Ebers, with the fragments of medical knowledge and practice in the Berlin and other papyri, contain but a slender body of information on pathological anatomy for a people with the unique opportunity of the Egyptians. In the five thousand years of shifting Egyptian dynasty before the Arabs swept across the banks of the Nile, some three quarters of a billion human bodies with all the ills to which the flesh is heir, passed under the hands of Egyptian embalmers. A large proportion of these were opened in the process, and countless thousands of diseased hearts, shrunken, abscessed and tuberculous lungs, cirrhotic livers, enlarged and atrophied spleens, infected kidneys and bowels, hardened arteries and clotted veins, in gigantic, solemn procession must have been seen, handled, and sealed in jars or thrown away by the despised "paraschistes," who made the initial incision, or the respected "taricheutes" who completed the evisceration. And of all the pathological knowledge that must have been occasionally if momentarily attained in these fifty centuries of monotonous and ruthless, coarse dissection, scarcely a trace has survived in written records.

It remained for modern anatomists to supply visible proof of the same vulnerability of internal human tissue forty centuries before Christ as today. From the brilliant investigations of Elliot Smith and Marc Ruffer on the mummies of ancient Egypt, we know that bone tumors and tuberculosis of the spine occurred, that osteomyelitis and arthritis deformans were common, that arteriosclerosis of the senile, atheromatous type with deposit of calcium salts, was at least as frequent as it is with us, and possibly more so, and that pneumonias, anthracosis, pleurisies, renal atrophies and abscesses, splenomegalies and gallstones troubled or cut off the Pharaohs and priests of Ammon, with the same kind of gross and microscopic change to be seen in the fresher human clay of the twentieth century.

Only with the Alexandrian Greeks of the last three centuries B.C., who were in Egypt, but not of it, did the civilization of the Nile make lasting contribution to the sciences of anatomy and pathology. To be sure, Greek students long before Hippocrates journeyed to Memphis and Heliopolis, and brought away much medical lore, but it was not pathology as the Greeks came to know it or as we know it today. The Greeks for all their polytheism were skeptical of the supernatural, and the highly speculative demonistic pathology of Egypt was less appealing than the still speculative but more rational humoralism of uncertain but probably Eastern origin, which finally became gospel among them.

The civilization of Mesopotamia contributed still less than Egypt of lasting value to pathology, and although the Code of Hammurabi (about 2200 B.C), and the clay tablet library of Assurbanipal in Nineveh (about 650 B.C.) give much information on medical and surgical practice among the Babylonians and Assyrians, they indicate that for the most part these peoples were content to assign disease of unobvious cause to malicious demonic influence.

The ancient Hebrews contributed independently to medical science in its sanitary and hygienic aspects, but accepted the theological conceptions of the Egyptians, Babylonians and Assyrians on the nature of disease. The Talmud, not completed until the second or third century A.D., had the benefit of matured Greek science, and reflects Greek ideas in recording superficial pathological anatomy. In the Talmud are recorded observations even in the field of experimental pathology, such as removal of the uterus and spleen. The careful proscriptions with regard to meat made the Jews familiar with pathological conditions in diseased animals, and no doubt in a subtle way went far to develop a pathologic anatomic tradition.

Assyrian, Babylonian, Jew and Egyptian alike went down before the Mede and Persian. But the Persians, who were to play such a great part in medicine in its period of Islamic domination, drew their medical science from alien sources in the pre-Christian era. Both Cyrus the Great and his son-in-law Darius I, who conquered Asia and Europe from the Indus to the Danube, called physicians to the Persian court from Egypt and Greece. It is even attested by Herodotus that Democedes of Crotona (520 B.C.), founder of a medical school in Athens, healed Darius' wife Atossa, daughter of Cyrus the Great, of a cancer of the breast. While the accuracy of the statement is questionable, the case is of interest to the pathologist as one of the first on record in tumor pathology.

In the brilliant period of Greek culture succeeding the ebb of Persian sway, fall the writings traditionally attributed to Hippocrates of Cos (460-370? B.C.), himself something of a mythical figure, but by age-long consent honored as the Father of Medicine. The uncertainties regarding the authorship of the great writings of the medical school of Cos are too well known to warrant repetition here. Modern scholarship is slowly achieving a separation of the "genuine" output of an individual Hip-

pocrates from the rest of the great body of medical doctrine
from the Coan school, but the sanction of tradition still warrants
our inclusion of the whole set of writings in the "Hippocratic
Collection."

With the Hippocratic group begins the scientific study of medicine and its divorce from theism and demonology. The lay sup-
plicants who placed clay models of cancerous breasts and
varicose veins on the temple altars assumed a supernatural cause
for their ills. The Hippocratic school, for their part, put their
stamp on a mechanistic conception of disease that soon dominated all medicine.

This was the humoral pathology. The origin of its underlying
doctrine is lost in antiquity. The theory probably came to the
Greeks through Babylon. In its simplest form it attributed
disease to anomalies of the fluids or humors of the body, and in
that form it persists today. The layman is still inclined to attribute boils to an effort of the blood to rid itself of its
impurities. But in the elaborate form of the Hippocratic school
the doctrine became a coil of complexity that even the generous
systematization of the modern, logic-loving historian cannot save
from seeming fantastic.

The humoral pathology developed by the school of Cos followed the example of philosophy in other fields in condensing
its unit elements to four. The four elements of Greek philosophy, air, water, fire and earth, and the four qualities, moisture,
cold, warmth and dryness, found their analogues in the four
humors of the body: the blood, which was warm and moist like
air; the phlegm, which was cold and moist like water; the yellow
bile, which was warm and dry like fire; and the black bile, which
was cold and dry like earth. The source of these humors was
fairly closely defined: for the blood, the heart; for the phlegm,
the brain; for the yellow bile, the liver; and for the black bile,
the spleen.

Health was believed to depend upon a normal blending or
εὐκρασία and disease upon a faulty mixture or δυσκρασία of the
humors. For example, an excess of phlegm in any part, dropping
down from the head, might result in the lungs in the characteristic signs of consumption, in the abdomen in dropsy, in the
bowels in dysentery, in the rectum in hemorrhoids, etc. Catarrh
and the supposed wide transportation of phlegm played an important part in Hippocratic pathogenesis. But it was the black
bile to which the ancients attributed the greatest power for
evil, and it is no exaggeration to term that stage of medical

PLATE I

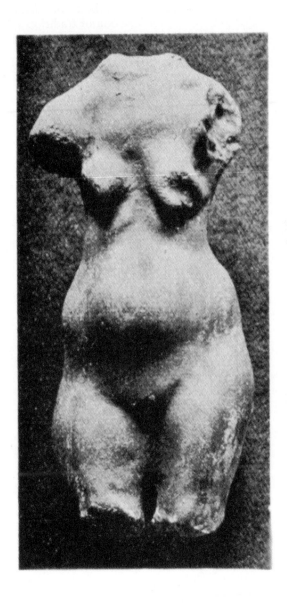

ANCIENT GREEK VOTIVE STATUETTE (ULCERATING
TUMOR OF THE BREAST)

history from Hippocrates to the Renaissance, the period of the *atra bilis.*

The character of the humoral dyscrasia determined the nature of the disease; the type of dyscrasia in turn was more or less dependent on the environment. Thus phlegmatic dyscrasias were common in winter, sanguinous in the spring, yellow bile aberrations in summer and black bile in the autumn. And thus were "epidemics" determined, the word in its original significance meaning general susceptibility to a given type of disease at a given place or time, more than spread of contagion. According to the Hippocratic concept, disease was prone to pass through three stages: a raw preliminary stage, a ripening stage, called the state of coction or pepsis, in which a cooking of the humors took place, and finally a stage of crisis, in which elimination of the superfluous humor or abnormal mixture of humors occurred.

According to this doctrine and the firmly grounded Hippocratic belief in the normal tendency of the body toward self cure, certain symptoms of disease, such as fever, represented the effort of the body to preserve life through coction or cooking of the altered fluids, while others, the cough, the vomiting, the diarrhoea, sweating, ulceration, etc., signified a crisis in which the excremental humors formed through the process of coction were expelled. Should the body be unable to accomplish coction or sustain crisis, the patient might die.

It is hard for us to see in this much besides fertile imagination, disregarding, as we do, the probability that science two thousand years hence will find much in our own medical and physiological belief just as fanciful. But the pathology of the Hippocratic school was not limited to speculation; there was much definite knowledge of disease processes to form a rational basis for medical practice.

The Hippocratic writers left good descriptions of inflammation in wounds, in puerperal sepsis, in pharyngitis, etc. They knew that patients with suppurative processes experienced chills and fevers. To be sure they considered pus merely transformed blood, heated to the point where it putrefied.

With cancer of superficial organs they were quite familiar. They introduced the terms καρκίνος and καρκίνωμα, carcinos apparently signifying a non-healing ulcer, even hemorrhoids, while carcinoma indicated a malignant tumor. A hard type of tumor, the σκίρρος, was distinguished from open carcinos or carcinoma. Our term scirrhus has almost the original signficance. In the

Diseases of Women scirrhous induration of the cervix of the uterus is mentioned, and lumps (φύματα) are described in the breasts, developing without ulceration into carcinos. Possibly the description referred to benign tumors.

The phymata of the ancients, mentioned as far back as Archilochus (719-633 B.C.), apparently included abscesses and tubercles as well as what we now consider true tumors. Frequent reference to phymata in the easily recognized descriptions of tuberculosis has led Flick to believe that the Hippocratic authors saw tubercles in the dead body, and associated them with lung disease. The Romans translated the word as "tubercle."

The descriptions of malaria are classic from the clinical point of view. Accounts which may refer to typhoid fever and influenza are less clear. Mumps was well described. Pneumonia was well known. The Hippocratic writers are often given great credit for distinguishing it from pleurisy, but what they described as pleurisy was probably truly pneumonia. Empyema is well described, as well as the spontaneous discharge of pus through the ribs and collapse of the lung.

The descriptions cover as a rule, however, only symptoms and external changes in the afflicted patient. With the exception of a few observations like the last, internal morbid anatomy was an unknown field. In the first place the Greeks of Hippocrates' time knew little normal anatomy. Renouard (Comiegny's translation) says, "Piecing together all the fragments of the Hippocratic writers relative to the structure of the human body, it would be impossible to compose from them a regular or complete treatise on anatomy, for with the exception of the skeleton they possessed very limited and imperfect notions of any organic apparatus. They confounded under a common name nerves, ligaments and tendons; they distinguished very imperfectly the arteries and veins, and the muscles in their eyes were inert masses designed solely to cover bones, serving as an envelope or ornament. They possessed in short only gross and false ideas on the structure and functions of the brain, heart, liver, lungs, digestive and generative apparatus, for the reason that they had never been able to devote themselves to regular dissections. But this did not prevent them from adducing very decided opinions on the organs and their functions, which no one could verify or deny."

For a proper appreciation of the obstacles to the development of an anatomical pathology, it must be recalled that the Greeks cremated their dead and that in popular superstition, without this conventional treatment of the departed, the soul continued to wander restlessly forever on the banks of the river Styx.

Nevertheless in the Hippocratic period the dissection of animals was assiduously cultivated and in a general way the position and character of the viscera were of course well known. Perhaps none added greater force to the movement than the unrivalled philosopher, physiologist, embryologist and comparative anatomist Aristotle (384-322 B.C.). This great scholar, while he never dissected human corpses himself, indirectly was of enormous influence on the science of anatomical dissection. His astonishingly extensive studies of animals and their development mark him as one of the founders of the science of zoölogy. He was the counselor of Philip of Macedon and tutor of Philip's son Alexander the Great. Among the several Alexandrias founded by the youthful empire builder was that at the mouth of the Nile, which became for a time the first city of the world. In the breakup of the Alexandrian empire, following the early death of the conqueror, this city and Egypt fell to Ptolemy of Macedonia, one of the most brilliant of Alexander's associates, himself influenced by Aristotle at the court of Philip.

Ptolemy, true to his intellectual training, established the Museum of Alexandria, the world's first university, and the great Alexandrian Library. His immediate successors added hugely to both. Here all branches of knowledge were cultivated, and none prospered more nor became more famous than the school of medicine. And here for the first time anatomy became the keystone for the structure of medical science. Here and apparently here only in the ancient world, dissection of the human body was practiced on an extensive scale. Both Celsus and Tertullian, indeed, claim that the early Alexandrian anatomists dissected living criminals. This is at least doubtful. It is said the Ptolemies themselves went into the dissection rooms and took part in the study of the dead, giving royal sanction to a process hitherto considered a desecration. And to Alexandria for four hundred years came the most promising medical students of the entire world.

Unfortunately the writings of the Alexandrian physicians are all lost. Our most important sources of information on their work are Celsus, and the Alexandrian students, particularly Galen. In anatomy two men stand out above all others, Herophilos and Erasistratos.

Herophilos, whose name is preserved for us in the "Torcular Herophili," was born at Chalcedon on the Bosphorus before

300 B.C., and became a pupil of Praxagoras of Cos, a disciple of the Hippocratic school noted for the extent to which he pushed the humoral theories of disease. Herophilos, however, although he followed the Hippocratic school in therapy, broke away from its speculative biology, and developed a physiological system of his own. He based life on four forces: a nourishing, located in the liver and digestive tract; a warming, located in the heart; a mental, located in the brain; and a sensitive, located in the nerves.

He was perhaps the first anatomist to pursue the science as an independent profession. So far from confining his attention to normal anatomy, however, he tried constantly to correlate it with disease, being, according to Pliny, "the first man who searched into the causes of disease" by dissection of the human body. We are quite ignorant, however, of what he learned, and can only guess at his contributions from the clear anatomical point of view of Celsus, who drew most of his pathological anatomy from "the Greeks," presumably meaning the Alexandrians.

His contemporary Erasistratos (about 310-250 B.C.) was more notable as a physiologist than an anatomist. He was born at Iulis on the island of Ceos, the son of a physician, and trained by Metrodorus, in turn a pupil of Chrysippos. The latter was one of the best known figures in the medical school of Cnidos, a rival school to that of Cos, and less inclined to abstract speculation. How long Erasistratos lived in Alexandria we do not know. For a time he was court physician at Antioch, capital of the Seleucid dynasty, another of the great sovereignties formed in the dissolution of Alexander's empire.

Erasistratos was truly one of the founders of pathology, although most of his exact concepts have long since been discarded. These were built on a system of physiology developed by himself, based on one of the most misleading scientific errors of the ancients. The arteries, as Erasistratos and his fellow dissectors saw them, were collapsed, containing at the most only air. Today we know that the elasticity of the arterial walls drives the blood on into the capillaries after death, and that air gets in only after the vessels are opened, an event inevitable in dissection. But Erasistratos knew nothing of capillaries, and believed in two circulations, one for blood from the heart and one for air from the lungs. These were the two important substances for the continuance of life, furnishing respectively nourishment and energy. The material distributed to the substance of the organs by the veins he called "parenchyma," a word we use today in a somewhat different sense. When the organs became overfilled, and the nutritive material was insufficiently digested, a condition of "plethora" developed.

He built his whole system of pathology around the condition of "plethora," localizing the disease anatomically, but explaining it in terms of this nutritional invention. And into the system he fitted easily as an example of *plethora* of the liver, his classic observation of dropsy of the abdominal cavity in the presence of woodeny hardness of the liver, or, as we would say, cirrhosis of the liver with ascites. And although the explanation of the accumulation of fluid in this familiar condition is different today, Erasistratos' definite association of the dropsy with the liver disease shines through the ages as a clear example of what the keen Alexandrian anatomists accomplished, for the first time in human history, by deliberate dissection for the purpose of explaining disease.

Inflammation was considered by Erasistratos to be the result of an overstuffing of the vessel terminals with blood. Fever was explained as an overfilling of the arteries with "pneuma" or air. Even the presence of blood in the arteries, which he considered normally air-containing, was pathological. One can see in his ideas a suggestion of our modern concept of hyperemia. Inflammation of the lungs was the result of a congestion of the lung arteries, arthritis a plethora of the joints. He was only making the same mistake that all morbid biologists of his time, and all subsequent time, have made, namely, confusion of cause and effect.

Both Herophilos and Erasistratos left an only slightly less brilliant group of followers, who like their masters cultivated anatomy and pathological anatomy, and thus broke far away from the *atra bilists* of the school of Cos. But the impetus given to medical science by the first Ptolemies was short-lived. Long before Julius Caesar annexed Egypt, Alexandrian science was conventionalized, pedantic and no longer productive. In 48 B.C. the great library was largely destroyed by Caesar's own soldiers. Fortunately before this happened much of the ancient learning of the medical Alexandrians had been transported in copied manuscripts to other lands, including Rome, where in the following century Celsus preserved the essence of it in the *De Re Medicina*.

Between the Alexandrians and Galen various more or less short-lived sects attempted to systematize diseases according to some simple formula. Asclepiades of Bithynia (about 128-56 B.C.) vigorously opposed the humoral pathology of Cos, and made just as little use of the learning of the Alexandrians. The essential teaching of Asclepiades was contained in the mechanistic doctrine of *"strictum et laxum,"* based on the supposed variability in tone of the innumerable body pores, hypothetical tubular spaces between the constituent and also hypothetical atoms of the body, through which the vital juices flowed. Undisturbed fluid motion, and corresponding health, depended on the maintenance of proper relation in size between the atoms and these pores. Were the latter unduly constricted or relaxed, disease resulted, acute as a rule in the former, chronic in the latter.

Asclepiades' disciple, Themison of Laodicea (123-43 B.C.), a bungler as a physician if we may judge from the biting comment of the caustic Juvenal, enlarged upon the *strictum et laxum* theory. Like Asclepiades he distinguished conditions characterized by (1) rigidity or tension and (2) relaxation, both dependent upon the state of the body pores, and associated with excess or deficiency of excretion. This he made the underlying basis for the school of methodism which he founded, and which was continued by his pupil Thessalos of Tralles. Many of the adherents of this school insisted that a knowledge of anatomy and its morbid changes was superfluous in the treatment of disease, a contention that doubtless had much to do with its eventual demise. Nevertheless methodism was in the ascendancy in Rome for the two centuries prior to the time of Galen, and far from defunct for a long period after that.

The pneumatic school, developed particularly by Athenaeus of Cilicia (about 70 B.C.) presupposed an aërial spirit or pneuma governing the solids and liquids of the body, the normal or abnormal action of which meant physiological or pathological phenomena. It contributed nothing and soon sank into insignificance as a school of thought, but its underlying doctrine has cropped out repeatedly from Galen to modern times, with the pneuma as the symbol of vitalism, an invisible prop on which Paracelsus, van Helmont and all the other mystics leaned heavily.

The greatest compilation of pathological knowledge before Galen is unquestionably the *De Re Medicina* of Cornelius Celsus, a Roman patrician of the time of Augustus and Tiberius (about 30 B.C. to 38 A.D.), apparently not a physician, but a man of leisure with comprehensive interest and a taste for literature. Probably because of his non-professional position, Celsus was ignored by or unknown to the medical profession of his day, and had absolutely no influence upon it. His works were soon lost, or buried in monasteries and only occasionally read, until 1443, when Thomas of Sarzana, afterwards Pope Nicholas V, ran across an ancient manuscript in the church of St. Ambrose in Milan, which was seized with eagerness by medical men of the time and exerted an enormous influence upon Renaissance medicine.

However little it influenced its own period, the *De Re Medicina* is interesting to us for the light it throws upon the state of knowledge of morbid anatomy and physiology available to the medical practitioner at the close of the pre-Christian era. Inspired chiefly by Hippocrates, the school of Asclepiades and the physician-anatomists of Alexandria, and based more directly, as it must have been, largely upon the other medical works now lost, it stands chiefly as the everlasting monument of the Alexandrian school, and in a sense, as Neuburger says, takes the place of their lost literature. It emphasizes, more than any other document, the enormous advance in anatomical point of view since Hippocrates.

Book IV of the eight books is a rich storehouse of pathological observation for its time, in which diseases are listed and described in the classic anatomical order, head, chest, abdomen, etc. Peripneumonia is described as a disease in which the whole lung is affected, obviously our pneumonia. Spleens so large as to be felt and firm enough to resist pressure, are recorded; certainly some of these were the result of malaria. There is mention of a "distemper seated in the large intestine principally affecting that part where I mentioned the caecum to be, accompanied by violent inflammation and vehement pains, particularly on the right side," and yet appendicitis did not enter the death records until after 1880!

Book III contains the classic definition of inflammation: *"Notae vero inflammationis sunt quatuor, rubor et tumor, cum calore et dolore,"* the redness, swelling, heat and pain that every medical student knows. In this same book is a clinical discussion of fevers, and a description of "that most dangerous kind of consumption, which the Greeks call φθίσις," with a strictly Hippocratic humoral explanation. Neither Celsus nor the Alexandrians could step quite clear of phlegm and the *atra bilis*.

The description of discharging "blood, sanies and pus" from wounds, in Book V, is classic, and the picture of skin cancer in the same book more than fair. His account of scrofula, "concretions of pus and blood, resembling small glands, growing chiefly in the neck but also in the armpits, groins and sides," brings up a familiar picture. The "collection tending entirely to suppuration, appropriating to itself the general name of abscess, red, hot and hard, changing to white when the suppuration is beginning, long after the onset of swelling and redness," leaves little to be desired for adequacy of description of the abscess.

Space does not permit more than mention of his account of gangrene of various parts, of "pus discharging from the ears, leading to insanity and death" (meningitis, unquestionably), and his description of gout, hernia, gonorrhoea and soft chancre, urinary calculi, etc. The eight books *De Re Medicina* may fitly be considered the first special pathology, a work almost modern, which, lacking the confusion and verbosity of Galen, stands as the only thing of its kind before the *Pathologiae Libri VII* of Jean Fernel.

PLATE II

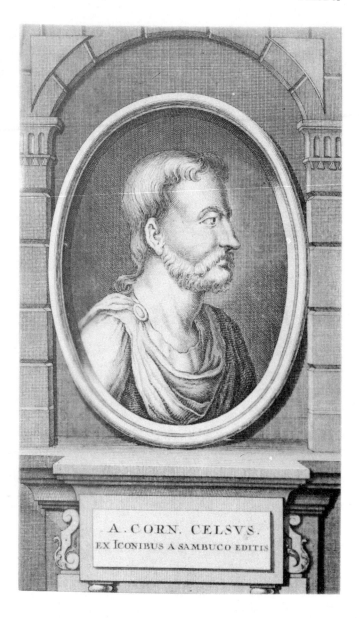

A. CORN. CELSVS.
EX ICONIBUS A SAMBUCO EDITIS

CORNELIUS CELSUS (ABOUT 30 B.C.-38 A.D.)

PLATE III

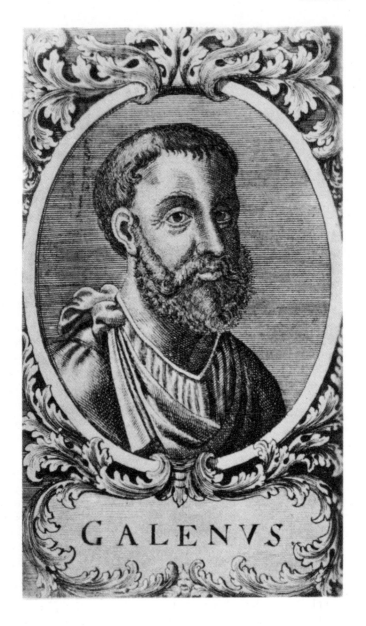

GALEN (129-201 A.D.)

CHAPTER II

Galen and the Middle Ages

With the opening of the Christian era the school of methodism was dominant in Rome, and disease commonly explained in terms of supposed variations in size, either constrictions or abnormal distentions, in the hypothetical pores of the body. The humoral pathology of Hippocrates and his associates and followers, was for the time in partial eclipse. The concrete observations of the Alexandrian anatomists on internal organic change in disease were largely neglected and in a fair way of being forgotten, although the knowledge was still available to the student who would read, and had been compiled in excellent, concise form by the Roman litterateur Celsus. The leading physicians were Asiatic Greeks, trained in abstract philosophy and good observers, but little inclined to submit their speculations to rigorous test. Human dissection had ceased to be practiced in the civilized world, and the science of pathological anatomy was therefore at a standstill.

Nevertheless there were many adherents of other sects, such as the pneumatists, who avoided both the humoral and the methodic pathological doctrine, and not a few unorthodox methodists, subscribing in a general way to the hypothesis of constricted and relaxed pores, but not hidebound, and open to truth regardless of its source. These are sometimes called eclectics. Of this group none achieved a greater reputation than Soranus (about 100 A.D.), a native of Ephesus in Asia Minor, a student in the later Alexandrian school of medicine, and finally practitioner during the reigns of Trajan and Hadrian in Rome. He is known chiefly for his development of obstetrics and gynecology, although he may have been equally capable in other branches of medicine, little more than his works on obstetrics and diseases of women having survived. He contributed to specific pathology mostly with respect to the female generative organs, leaving descriptions of inflammation of the uterus, scirrhous tumors and "scleromata" of the uterus (possibly cancer and our benign "fibroid" tumors), and the less serious displacements, and leucorrhoea and excessive bleeding. Through the methodist compiler and systematist Caelius Aurelianus we know something of his general pathology, which was methodist in type, emphasizing the supposed general state of the body as well as any particular anatomical manifestations. Pneumonia, for example, was considered a generalized disease, with a tendency toward specific pulmonary localization.

Rufus of Ephesus, also educated in Alexandria, and a contemporary of Soranus in Rome, left good descriptions of two of the great plagues of increasing seriousness in the West, leprosy and bubonic plague, as well as of erysipelas. His anatomical point of view is illustrated in his little book of nomenclature *On the Naming of the Parts of the Human Body*, and it is noteworthy that he lamented his lack of opportunity to dissect bodies of men, as was formerly done, and his own restriction to monkeys. He described skin cancer, and some of his records are supposed to refer to melanotic tumors.

One of the greatest surgeons of the time was another contemporary of Soranus, a Syrian, Archigenes of Apameia, who is usually considered a representative of the pneumatic school. We are uncertain just what he wrote, but have good reason to believe that much of the writings of Aretaeus and Aëtius are based largely on Archigenes, the ancients having a notorious habit of incorporating vast treatises of others into their own works without even perfunctory thanks. Archigenes seems to have known a good deal about cancer of the breast and uterus, and recognized the occasional occurrence of cancer in the breasts of men. He repeated the analogy to the tenacious hold of the crab, which had impressed the early Greeks, and recognizing the usual futility of surgical removal, left a salve, the *medicamentum Archigenis ad cancros ulceratos*, in use to the sixteenth century.

The eclectic pneumatist Aretaeus of Cappadocia, whose exact period is still conjectural, left a classic on *The Causes and Characteristics of Acute and Chronic Disease* which is Hippocratic in its general physiology and pathological doctrine, but far more modern in its attention to anatomical detail. Each chapter opens with a short anatomical description of the part treated. For each disease he at least presumed an anatomical basis, and his belief in the presence of ulcers of the intestine in dysentery and explanation of crossed paralysis, his correlation of ascites and general anasarca with dyspnoea and a failing heart action, and his picture of a "lung not decayed, but filled with humors and concretions" in phthisis, with reference to the usual terminal looseness of the bowels, and truly appalling picture of the associated emaciation, indicate a predominately anatomical point of view. His clinical accounts of·pneumonia, diabetes, leprosy and diphtheria (*ulcera Syriaca*) have been much praised. Much of the information, according to Wellmann, must have come from Archigenes, but the teaching method is presumably Aretaeus' own. He quotes only Hippocrates, and initiates the return to humoral explanation of disease that culminated with Galen.

Galen (129-201 A.D.) was born in the rich and cultured city of Pergamus, Asia Minor. Before he was twenty he was off on those travels that took him to most of the medical centers of the civilized world. Alexandria was his ultimate goal, however, and it was Alexandria to which he referred most in later years. There he was a pupil of the school developed by the anatomist Marinos, a man well versed in the teaching of his celebrated predecessors, who claimed to have verified all their discoveries in the human body with his own hands.

At twenty-eight he was back in Pergamus, and, already known through his writings as a rising young anatomist, was appointed physician to the gladiators, a position affording much surgical experience. After four years this palled and he set out, like so many of the brilliant young physicians of Asia Minor, for Rome, where he spent five years practicing medicine and holding anatomical discourses before select audiences, never for a moment, however, despite his popularity, giving up his anatomical research. These five Roman years were among his best.

The professional jealousy of his fellow physicians ultimately, however, made Rome unpleasant for him. Galen published his opinion of his opponents in scathing terms, but left town none the less, just escaping a visitation of the plague in 166 A.D. He had no sooner reached Pergamus than he received a summons from the Roman Emperor Marcus Aurelius Antoninus to join him and Verus in Aquileia, where war was being prepared against the Teutonic tribe of Marcomanni and Quadi. Galen disliked the prospect, but bowed to the command, proceeding through Thrace and Macedonia, only to see the military project utterly upset by another outbreak of plague, in which Verus died. Galen trailed after Antoninus to Rome, to let him know quite definitely that he had had enough of the field, and that his domain was quiet practice and scholarly research. Antoninus acquiesced, appointing him personal physician to his son Commodus, a position making no great demands on Galen's time, and from 169 A.D. to the end of his life, under Antoninus, Commodus and Septimius Severus, the industrious physician devoted practically undisturbed attention to scientific work and voluminous writing, not only on medicine in all its phases, but even on philosophy and rhetoric.

Galen is perhaps the greatest medical figure of all time. He has been much abused because his works held despotic authority over European medicine for thirteen centuries after his death, with all their error as well as truth accepted as medical gospel. It is hard to see how this is Galen's fault. It is true that he rated himself high, and that his works teem with hearty expressions of self-approbation and equally and unmistakable disapproval of those with whom he disagreed. This does not seem to have been professional bad form in the second century, however.

Galen's preëminence rests first of all on his indefatigable industry and enormous productivity. His mistakes and false analogies do not neutralize the progress he made, any more than the unquestionably numerous mistakes daily broadcast in the scientific literature of the twentieth century, will in the end nullify this century's scientific progress. The twenty-first will presumably preserve the good and discard the false, just as Vesalius, Colombo, Fallopius, Harvey and Morgagni did with the works of Galen, leaving, let it be understood, an enormous body of established fact.

We are not concerned here with Galen's anatomical and physiological beliefs and discoveries, except as they bear on his contributions to pathology. Galen's general pathology was the now quite defunct humoral doctrine of the Hippocratic collection, supplemented by his own conception of a guiding spirit or pneuma; and it must be admitted that he outhumored the most extravagant humoralists of the school of Cos. It was Galen more than Hippocrates who made the Middle Ages thirteen centuries of dread of the *atra bilis*. It was, however, Galen's enormous specific knowledge of disease, i.e., his special pathology, that stamped his whole output, including his humoral pathology, with authority.

We must remember that Galen's knowledge of morbid change in the body was accumulated without the opportunity for postmortem examination. After he left Alexandria he dissected not more than two or three human bodies, although he perhaps saw a few presumably normal bodies of slain barbarians opened by the military surgeons in his brief service with the legions. He was forced to snatch the opportunity of improving his knowledge of the anatomic basis of disease from the living patient, and by shrewd combination of his knowledge of the anatomy of apes and swine, and his familiarity with external lesions in man, guess at the specific internal abnormalities. Had Roman tradition licensed necropsy there is no limit to what he might have learned. No man who ever lived would have made more of the opportunity.

Galen's views and discoveries in pathology are found largely in his *Seats of Disease,* his *Abnormal Tumors,* the *Therapeutic Method—addressed to Glaucon,* his work on the *Natural Faculties,* and that on *Parts Affected.* The first is a large treatise on local pathology and diagnosis. The work on tumors is brief, but important. The *Therapeutic Method,* addressed to a philosopher friend, is a large work describing the nature of individual diseases and their treatment. It is at once a textbook of pathology and of therapeutics. The *Natural Faculties* is a physiological text, with frequent reference to the abnormal, and the *Parts Affected,* as the name indicates, really a great reference book of special pathology and pathological physiology.

Much of Galen's pathogenesis is based on his conception of presentation (πρόσθεσις) and adhesion (πρόσφυσις). When a proper amount of the right kind of fluid reached a given organ it adhered and was there utilized. Normal digestion and absorption of fluid from the intestine is a simple illustration. Should an imbalance, however, occur between presentation and adhesion, disease resulted. If the alimentary tract, for example, refused to accept the food presented, i.e., failed to permit adhesion, vomiting occurred.

Such was his explanation, likewise, for edema, and its generalized form anasarca, in which the body cavities and subcutaneous tissue are filled with fluid, a condition with which Galen was doubtless as familiar in its gross, external aspects as we are. To Galen the water-logging of the tissue occurred because the fluid presented to the parts was too watery, failed to adhere and become converted into a tissue juice, and therefore easily slipped away from the solid parts of the body. It must be remembered that the explanations of edema today are still speculative.

He made a bad error in refuting Erasistratos' explanation of ascites or accumulation of fluid in the abdominal cavity. The Alexandrian had recorded this condition as the result of a woodeny hardness of the liver, "cirrhosis," as we say today (Chapter I). Apparently anything Erasistratos said was to Galen like a red rag to a bull, and he felt forced to charge it. In discussing abdominal dropsy Galen wrote that he had frequently seen it produced by the simple suppression (cauterization?) of hemorrhoids, and adds, "certainly the liver was not implicated in that kind of dropsy." As a matter of fact it probably was, for, as we know today, the distended hemorrhoidal veins might well have owed their enlarged, incommodious state to the fact that they were taking over one of the functions of the liver, viz., passage of blood from the intestinal venous system to the general circulation. Great enlargement of the hemorrhoidal veins might furnish sufficient compensation for a disordered liver, and ascites be avoided. Galen's "suppression" of the hemorrhoids simply destroyed the compensation. In general all of Galen's explanations of changes due to circulatory abnormalities suffered from his faulty knowledge of the blood circulation.

Jaundice was explained on a basis similar to edema. Galen was quite well aware that jaundice is the result of absorption of bile into the blood, and familiar with the fact that when the body is full of bile the stools are frequently free from it. He missed the connection, however, and fell back for his explanation of jaundice upon the ancient supposition of relation between the spleen and bile. But whereas the school of Cos believed that jaundice resulted from excessive secretion of bile by the spleen, Galen proposed the theory that it was due to a failure of the spleen to remove the black bile already present in the blood. Here again was a disbalance between presentation and adhesion. The rôle of the spleen was to clear the blood of black bile, but if the spleen was out of order, enlarged, for example, as he says, from internal suppuration, in spite of normal presentation adherence might fail to occur, and the blood, therefore, take on a bad color. This was an ingenious enough theory for the second century A.D., no different in character from the twentieth-century hypothesis of a detoxicating function in the liver and thyroid; no doubt the anatomical basis for it was Galen's observation of jaundice in the presence of an enlarged, that is palpable, and therefore diseased spleen, not an infrequent occurrence.

Galen was a keen student of inflammation. He included it among the morbid swellings or tumors, was laborious and long-winded in his explanation, and piercing in his apprehension of fact. In accordance with his general theory of disease as an alteration in the humors or their *pneumatic* control, he considered inflammation to be due to an excessive accumulation of any of these in the affected part. With continued stagnation of the humors arose the four cardinal symptoms of redness, swelling, pain, and heat, to which he added a fifth, pulsation. After these came exudation of serum (ἴχωρ) and suppuration, possibly followed by general corruption (σῆψις). Gangrene was an inflammation of great extent, and Galen was acute enough to note that in this condition in the legs, the arteries were impermeable.

Had Galen stopped there, much good and no harm might have resulted, but his insistence on the full measure of the humoral doctrine led to far reaching mischief. A too literal disciple of his master Hippocrates in this instance, he emphasized "coction" or suppuration as an essential part in the healing of wounds, to such a degree that his slavish apostles of later centuries, particularly the Arabs, instead of letting nature take its course in this respect, as did Hippocrates and Galen, went to all lengths to promote suppuration, and with them arose the notion of "laudable pus," the most pernicious concept that ever sullied medicine.

On the other hand Galen's shrewd reasoning from external signs concerning internal inflammations was at times superb. He was not only able to detect pus in the urine, but from its state made skillful deductions as to its origin. If it was in coarse suspension or membranous flakes, he assumed, probably correctly, that it came from the bladder. If it was intimately mixed with the urine he believed it came from the kidney or ureter.

Galen was familiar with the major facts of urinary secretion, largely through his masterly experiments on the kidneys of living animals. He distinguished somewhat vaguely inflammations of the kidney (νεφρῖτις) with increased and decreased output of urine, but was more familiar with the kind of kidney inflammation associated with the presence of calculi. He knew that stones found in the bladder often came from the kidney, and might occasion terrific pain in their passage through the ureter. He recognized a similarity between urinary calculi and gouty deposits in joints.

In pulmonary pathology he made less advance, although he wrote voluminously. Bronchitis he knew well. He had all the knowledge of antiquity on empyema, which he included among the morbid swellings. He made the usual classic distinction between peripneumonia and pleuritis, like all the ancients overemphasizing pleuritis as an entity. On phthisis he copied the

Hippocratic writers. Unfortunately he tells us nothing of its prevalence in Rome, simply stating that it was commoner in women than men. The cause was acrid phlegm dropping down from the brain, the old Hippocratic notion, or more commonly hemorrhage in the lung, the eternal confusion of cause and effect. The hemorrhage he considered the result of traumatic rupture of blood vessels in the lung, or of local ulceration. He recognized chronic ulceration of the lung, with occasional coughing even of pieces of lung and small stones. This was phthisis if associated with profound emaciation, otherwise not.

Galen copied what the Greeks had to say about phymata or tubercles, apparently without either seeing them or understanding them. Nevertheless he felt qualified to explain them, and attributed their presence to a coagulation making the juices too thick to pass through the veins. His conception of tuberculosis was thus vague and highly confused, an illustration of the utter hopelessness of its understanding without post-mortem examination. And it is noteworthy that no further light was thrown on the disease until Sylvius (de le Boë) studied the dead bodies of consumptives—fifteen centuries later.

Galen made an elaborate symptomatic classification of fevers, for which he gave a futile, speculative humoral etiology. He distinguished well the continuous from the intermittent fever, and credited phlegm, yellow bile and the *atra bilis* with special rôles in the quotidian, tertian and quartan forms of intermittent (or malarial) fever. The Roman marshes must have furnished Galen unlimited opportunity for the clinical study of malaria.

His discussion of tumors is of exceptional interest in that his classification, in its Latin translation, was followed until long after the Renaissance. Three great groups were distinguished: the *tumores secundum naturam,* which included all normal physiological swellings, such as the breasts at puberty and the gravid uterus; the *tumores supra naturam,* i.e., the productive processes following injury, such as callus formation after fracture; and the great group of *tumores praeter naturam,* which included the neoplasms, or our true tumors, as well as many inflammatory lesions, localized edemas, gangrene, cysts and other affections, the true nature of which Galen could not determine. The scirrhus, carcinos and carcinoma of the ancient Greeks reappear, with malignancy distinguished more or less definitely on the basis of ulceration. The black bile was the cause of all cancer. Galen claimed to have observed repeatedly that melancholic women were more prone to carcinoma than those of sanguine temperament, and the regions where in his opinion the black bile thickened, viz., the face, lips and breast, were most liable to the development of the tumor. The malignant ulcerating form was due to an acrid bile, while a milder bile produced the cancer occultus, i.e., non-ulcerated cancer. He had no knowledge of internal cancer, and no suspicion of the phenomenon of metastasis. The Hippocratic analogy of cancer with the crab, which led to both terms καρκίνος and *cancer,* is repeated by Galen: "Just as in a crab feet extend from every part of the body, so in this disease the veins are distended forming a figure quite similar." Galen had no knowledge of the lymphatics, and what we now know to be extensions into the lymph channels were to him simply growths into the veins, forming a ready contact between the tumor mass and the *atra bilis.* The distended vessels in the neighborhood of the swelling formed part of his picture of a crab-like mass.

Such, in brief, was the pathology of Galen, supreme for a thousand years. The wise and great Pergamene had rung the knell on methodism, revivified the Alexandrian anatomical idea of disease, and restored in a most extraordinary fashion the humoral etiological theories of the school of Hippocrates. It was not so much these achievements, however, that led to Galen's age-long domination of medicine, as his bold and largely successful attempt to make a unified science of biology, with separate branches of anatomy, physiology, and pathology, the latter characterized by specific underlying *diatheses,* each with its essential πάθος, or disturbance of vital process. The central idea of Galen's physiology, viz., teleology, unmistakably delineated in his immortal physiological text *On the Use of Parts,* expressing the great idea of design in nature, conformed perfectly with the rising tide of monotheism, and Christian and Moslem alike asked nothing better.

With the passing of Galen medicine entered its long period of unproductivity. The Romans, with the exception of Celsus, contributed nothing to the advance of medical knowledge, and with the incursions of barbarians from the North and the increasing turbulence of life in Rome, the Greek physicians from Asia Minor and the islands found the Western capital less and less conducive to scholarly existence. Even at the quieter court of the Eastern Empire at Byzantium, or Constantinople, the true spirit of inquiry was in abeyance and the best of the Greek scholars contented themselves with editing and revising the works of the ancients, Hippocrates, Archigenes, Antyllus, Soranus, Galen, etc.

Four names stand out preëminently in this Byzantine period of compilation, Oribasius, Aëtius, Alexander of Tralles and Paul of Aegina. Oribasius (325-403), a native, like Galen, of Pergamus, became physician to the Emperor Julian surnamed the Apostate, at whose court he had the leisure and opportunity of studying and bringing up to date the works of many of the older writers. His own works, consisting originally of seventy books, of which only twenty-five are extant, have the great merit of quotation with the author's name mentioned. Through Oribasius the works of Archigenes, Antyllus and others were preserved for posterity.

Aëtius of Amida in Mesopotamia (502-575) was physician to the Emperor Justinian. His work is largely compiled from the writings of Rufus of Ephesus, Leonides of Alexandria, Soranus and Archigenes. He gave an excellent description of carcinoma of the uterus, distinguishing ulcerated and non-ulcerated forms. The tumor was usually at the cervix, hard, resistant and uneven to the touch, and reddish, almost livid. From it came a thin, watery, reddish yellow discharge. He considered it a quite incurable condition. He probably derived his knowledge of this cancer from Archigenes. He also, as Wolff brings out, describes fissures, nodules and condylomas in the region of the anus in such a way as to suggest carcinoma of the rectum. Aëtius' work is considered by Garrison to contain the best account of disease of the eye, ear, nose, throat and teeth in antiquity. Except in surgery, however, Aëtius showed little originality or fresh observation, and it cannot be said that he added anything of note to pathology.

Alexander of Tralles (525-605), a student in many lands, who lived for a time both in Rome and Byzantium, is noted for his correlation of physical diagnosis and pathological anatomy. His diagnoses of ascites by percussion, of edema by pitting, and large spleen by palpation, were no doubt, as Allbutt points out, part of the current medical knowledge of the time, and show that in spite of the continued dominance of the humoral doctrines of etiology the notion of an anatomical basis was becoming more and more firmly grounded.

Paul of Aegina (625-690) wrote an *Epitome* of medicine of great and lasting influence, particularly in surgery, greatly extending the writings of Oribasius. How much original observation should be credited to Paul is doubtful. It is noteworthy that somewhere between Galen's time and that of Alexander of

Tralles and Paul the existence of internal cancer had been recognized. Alexander mentions cancer of the liver, and Paul says: *"In omni corporis parte cancer nasci solet."* He was a docile *atra bilist,* however, and added nothing to the theory of pathology. And with him closes the productive period of Byzantine medical scholarship, even in the field of compilation. The future lay with the Arab.

It is worth while to note how this came about. Early in the seventh century a nomadic people in the Arabian desert and quiet town-folk in the desert cities of Medina and Mecca had accepted a new Prophet, and once more with visions of world subjugation conquering armies were loose between Mesopotamia and the Nile. Under the Prophet's successors, Moslem soldiers overran Syria, and most of Byzantine Asia Minor and Persia. Egypt collapsed without a struggle and hosts of Saracen cavalry surged across North Africa. Eventually they crossed the Strait of Gibraltar, conquered Spain and reached the Pyrenees. They were even pushing into France when finally, a century to the year after the Prophet Mohammed died, Charles Martel and his Frankish troops administered their first crushing defeat in the West. The tide rolled back and war-like Saracens never again crossed the Pyrenees, but from Spain to the eastern limits of Turkestan across Africa and Asia Minor there remained an unbroken belt of Moslem power.

And then, strangely, out of the raiding, pillaging, destroying Islamites developed a gentle race with more than a fair share of quiet scholars. Even the despised Jew, uneasy, uncertain of his future in all the rest of Europe, was given asylum and the opportunity to develop his talents. And between them the Moslem and the Jew for three hundred years furnished the light and talent of medicine.

The Arabs had acquired their first contact with the best medical thought of the day at the time of their Persian conquest. In Persia was a great medical school founded by the well educated Nestorian Greeks, a Christian sect, forced out of their homes in Byzantine lands by the emperor Justinian. By this curious link medical leadership passed from Constantinople to Bagdad.

Two of the greatest medical writers of the Islamic period were Persians, Rhazes and Avicenna. Rhazes (860-932), trained in medicine in Bagdad, was the author of the *Continens,* a comprehensive work in Arabic, the *Almansur,* a briefer work, and a treatise on smallpox and measles, containing the first clear-cut description of these diseases. In thought and practice Rhazes was a follower of Galen and Hippocrates.

The other Persian, Avicenna of Bokhara and Bagdad (980-1037), was an illustrious physician, dissipated but brilliant, whose major work, the *Canon,* all but achieved the impossible of supplanting Galen. Up to the fifteenth century it was the best single work in medicine. In general, however, it was merely a compilation, resting heavily on the doctrines of Galen and philosophy of Aristotle. The original material of chief note is, like that of Rhazes, in the field of the eruptive fevers.

Avicenna's ideas furnish an interesting light on the extent of smallpox among his people. The human race appeared to him so nearly universally afflicted with this disease that he came to think of it as the inherent lot of mankind, each individual contracting it in the womb of his mother. An orthodox humoralist, he considered the eruption a synergy of vital forces for the purpose of removing the offending fluid.

In the Western Caliphate, Avenzoar (1070-1162), a highly educated Jewish physician of cultured family, born near Seville, practiced medicine at the court of Cordova. He is of especial interest in pathology because he knew of carcinoma of the esophagus and carcinoma of the stomach. His description of cancer of the stomach (*verruca ventriculi,* wart of the stomach), is a clear-cut clinical account of a common condition, which curiously enough escaped anatomical understanding up to the time of Benivieni. The description of carcinoma of the esophagus is unmistakable, a condition "beginning with mild pain and difficulty in swallowing, and going on gradually to its complete prevention." Avenzoar passed silver sounds in cancer of the esophagus, and used nutritive enemas in both the stomach and esophageal tumors. He also described serous pericarditis and was the first to describe the mite of scabies, being entitled in the opinion of Garrison to be considered the first parasitologist after Alexander of Tralles.

On the whole, however, the Arabian school, like the Byzantine copyists, did little to advance the understanding of the nature of disease or science of pathology except in connection with the exanthemata. From our point of view the Moslems were hopelessly handicapped by the Koran's prohibition of dissection or other mutilation of the dead, a curious paradox when we recall some of the mutilations of the living credited to the pillaging Arabs. Their great field was pharmacy, and while they pushed this to the point where it was worse than fantastic, they made contributions of lasting value in its parent science, chemistry.

With the decline of Arabian medicine after the Crusades, continental monasteries, from the twelfth to fifteenth centuries, became chiefly responsible for keeping Greek medicine alive. Monks became physicians, although not surgeons, and the quieter ones among them, who flinched most from the more favored, boisterous, military career of the age, occupied themselves with copying and annotating ancient manuscripts, particularly Galen. The forgotten work of Celsus also was kept alive through this medium. It was at first a sterile time as regards medical advance, but an awakening gradually became apparent in the development of the universities, Montpellier, and Paris, and particularly the Italian schools, Salerno, Bologna, and Padua. While Salerno, with its unique medical relation to the Crusades, came to excel in practical surgery, in Bologna a new interest awoke in the fundamental sciences, anatomy and pathological anatomy.

To Bologna in 1260, already an enormous school, with 10,000 students from all parts of Europe, came Taddeo di Alderotto. His influence had much to do with the sustained high position of Bolognese medicine. Apparently he was the first to make dissections of the human body a regular part of university teaching. We have no exact information to prove this, but references to dissections in the writings of his pupils Bartolomeo da Varignana (died 1318), Henri de Mondeville (died 1320) and Mondino de' Luzzi (died 1326) suggest it.

Good evidence has been adduced by Singer that the first openings of the human body in this period were necropsies, for clues to the cause of disease or for judicial reasons, rather than dissections for anatomical information. Strange as it may seem, in the revival of learning at the Italian universities, the scientific study of pathological anatomy commenced before the study of the normal, and ultimately gave the necessary stimulus to the latter. The reason for this, however, is fairly simple. Normal anatomy was supposed to be established, in the works of the incomparable Galen and his brilliant copier Avicenna, whose *Canon* had been recently translated into Latin.

Bodies had frequently been opened to determine the cause of the plague, as early as the sixth century in Byzantium, according to Morgagni, but the results of these necropsies have not come down to us. One of the first records of a legal post-mortem is of that performed on the body of a certain nobleman named

Azzolino, who died in 1302 under circumstances suggesting poisoning, a suspicion only too reasonably attached to sudden deaths in general in Italy in medieval and Renaissance times. In this case a post-mortem was ordered by court, and performed by a committee under the direction of Bartolomeo da Varignana, the pupil of Taddeo. Their decision is not clear, but their report, which still survives, makes it certain that the body was opened and examined.

A medico-legal post-mortem is also credited to William of Saliceto (about 1201-1280), an able Bolognese surgeon and contemporary of Taddeo, who seems to have had considerable interest in pathological anatomy. Apparently it was not an uncommon practice. William's post-mortem investigation may have been the source of his well known reference to *"durities renum,"* which has been interpreted as the earliest reference extant to the pathological anatomy of Bright's disease. This occurs in his *Summa Conservationum* (1275), the first book of which is a veritable special pathology, in which abnormalities of the organs from the head to the feet are considered. The reference is too vague to be of much significance, but it is interesting that he correlated kidney disease with the onset of dropsy.

Plate IV shows one of the earliest known illustrations of a post-mortem examination, taken from a manuscript which Dr. Singer dates in the first half of the fourteenth century.

There has been much discussion concerning theological proscription and the return to dissection. Frederick II (1194-1250), Holy Roman Emperor, crusader and self-crowned King of Jerusalem, one of the most enlightened men of his age and founder of the University of Naples, is credited with the first law authorizing human dissection. Yet long after 1300 most people in Europe were probably still thoroughly imbued with the idea that dissecting a corpse was a desecration. The famous Bull *De Sepulturis* of Pope Boniface VIII (1300) has been held responsible for much of this attitude toward dissection. This read, "Persons cutting up bodies of the dead and barbarously cooking them, in order to separate the bones from the flesh for transportation and burial in their own country, are by that act excommunicated." However it came to be interpreted in later years, originally the bull was directed purely against a common practice of the Crusaders. The remains of many noted knights of the cross returned to Europe in this fashion.

It is nevertheless true that the question of sinfulness in dissection was finally referred to a churchly authority for an opin-

PLATE IV

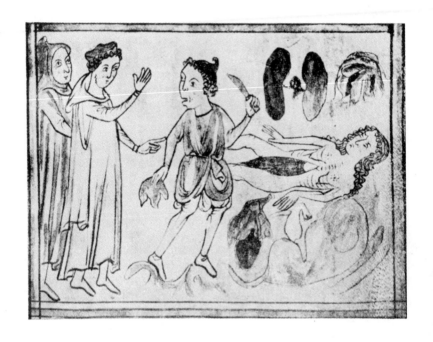

NECROPSY SCENE FROM THE FOURTEENTH CENTURY
Reproduced from a MS in the Bodleian Library through the
courtesy of Dr. Charles Singer

ion. Because of many complaints concerning the increase in dissection, Charles V, in 1556, laid the matter before the theological faculty of the University of Salamanca. These wise and broad-minded theologians concluded that "the dissection of human corpses serves a useful purpose, and is therefore permissible to Christians of the Catholic Church," a decision probably of much weight in ensuing years.

With the rise of the Italian universities apparently a rivalry developed which favored the progress of anatomical science. Whereas at first the material for anatomical study was obtained through clandestine grave robbing by irreverent medical students, and the unpleasant practice, at the best, winked at by the authorities, after 1360 municipal legislators saw the wisdom of favoring dissection, just as they promoted other sciences or anything else that increased the local reputation. Executed criminals furnished the necessary material, their forfeiture of mortal rights thus being extended beyond death.

Returning to the school of Taddeo, we find that one of his pupils, Mondino (1275-1326?), came to rival Galen as an authority on anatomy. He succeeded his master as the leading anatomist of the Bologna school, and in 1316 wrote a book, apparently based on Galen, the Arabians and a few bodies he dissected himself, which for two hundred years was the standard text, and even legally so designated. In it are recorded the results of two post-mortems of 1315 on female cadavers, in which he attempted to determine the effect of pregnancy on the subsequent size of the uterus. Early in the sixteenth century, the famous anatomist Marcantonio della Torre, who with the assistance of Leonardo da Vinci was in a fair way to anticipate Vesalius, before his untimely death, was obliged to petition the authorities in his desire to substitute Galen in the original for Mondino in his teaching.

Another pupil of Taddeo, the surgeon Henri de Mondeville (about 1250-1320), who was teaching in Montpellier while Mondino occupied the chair of anatomy in Bologna, is particularly noteworthy to the pathologist and surgeon for his insistence on cleanliness in operation and opposition to the common surgical practice of inducing suppuration as an adjunct to wound healing. Henri wrote a great surgery, which was supplanted, however, in the next generation by the famous *Magna Chirurgia* of Guy de Chauliac (1300-1370). Henri was a good surgeon but a Galenist in theory, explaining the localization of cancer in glands, for example, on the ground that "the melancholic material enters more easily a spongy than solid place."

Guy de Chauliac also followed the views of Galen and Avicenna. Unlike Henri, he believed in "laudable pus" and the conventional theory of coction and expulsion of irritant humors through suppuration in the healing of wounds. Guy followed a classification of "abscesses" which has some points of contact with modern knowledge, and which became conventional in the late Middle Ages. Abscesses were of two kinds: (1) hot, like phlegmon, pustules, gangrene and anthrax, and (2) cold, like scrofula, dropsy, tympanites and cancer. The term thus included all swellings, but had the merit of including the acute inflammatory swellings in a special group almost synonymous with our abscess.

Guy lived through two visitations of the plague while he was physician to the popes in Avignon, caught the disease himself and left a good description of it. He also wrote an excellent account of leprosy, at that time endemic through all Europe. He was a thorough Galenist as regards cancer.

Throughout the fourteenth and fifteenth centuries dissections for teaching, mostly just to substantiate Galen and Mondino, became increasingly common. Could they have been conducted in a more leisurely manner, a good deal of new knowledge of pathological anatomy might have accumulated. But bodies putrefied rapidly, and it was customary to push through the job in four hasty sessions. The parts were pointed out by an assistant while the professor monotonously droned out Galen without paying much attention to the subject on the table below him, and there was little time for studying abnormalities. Nevertheless the anatomical idea was steadily gaining ground, and occasionally someone commented on the internal lesions, like Pietro di Montagnana (died 1460), who claimed to have seen diseased hearts in the course of fourteen post-mortem examinations and dissections made in Padua.

CHAPTER III

The Pathology of the Renaissance

The revival of learning, which brought back the old classics just in time to meet the printing press, and opened up the world for Christopher Columbus, Luther, Copernicus and Vesalius, carried in the humble beginnings of pathological anatomy too, as a separate science.

We have seen how the study of normal human anatomy came to be recognized as worthwhile in the rising universities of the twelfth to fifteenth centuries, but moped in the spell of Galen's authority. That anatomical changes were associated with disease was of course obvious, and Galen had systematized them to a degree little appreciated today. Yet little attention was focused on them, except in their surgical aspects, and the explanations of disease which were good enough for Hippocrates, Galen and the Arabian masters satisfied the best thinkers in the new medical schools.

Naturally there were independent minds too, as in all ages, and the new liberty gave them opportunity. In the city of Florence in the colorful time of Lorenzo de' Medici and Machiavelli, one Antonio Benivieni (about 1443 to 1502), a practicing physician, blazed the new trail. Perhaps it is only through the coincidence of printing that he has this distinction, but more probably it was the combination of a fresh thinker and a cordial age.

He was born in Florence, a member of an ancient and noble Florentine family. Educated in the Universities of Pisa and Siena, he practiced medicine in his native city for more than thirty years. We would not know much about his life if his brother Geronimo in 1507, five years after Antonio's death, had not collected his case records, apparently quite carefully kept, and with the encouragement of Jean Rosatus, a distinguished physician and old friend of the practicing Benivieni, published them in book form. The title of this little classic is *De Abditis Nonnullis ac Mirandis Morborum et Sanationum Causis.* Note the *"abditis."* For the first time since the days of Erasistratos, physicians were unconcernedly and routinely searching out the *hidden* or internal causes of symptoms as revealed by necropsy. The revelations of twenty post-mortem examinations, performed by Benivieni himself or his friends, are included in the one hundred and eleven short chapters of the book.

The opening chapter is on the *Morbus Gallicus.* Syphilis, too, came with the Renaissance. Benivieni's life was drawing short as this new scourge was speeding across Europe, but he evidently saw much of it in his closing years, and described its superficial manifestations well, including the skull erosions, which seem to have been more common then than now.

But the cream of the work is the post-mortem observation. Benivieni was the first physician to our knowledge to request permission of his patient's relatives to perform necropsies in obscure cases, and has frequently been called the father of pathological anatomy in our curious and mistaken tendency to assign sudden paternity to each science.

After all, he left little ground work for establishing a science, and was enough a product of his time to believe in obsession by demons, and not to go beyond Galen in his citation of scientific authority. Nor can it be said that he had much influence upon the scientific thought of his successors, although they all quoted him. His great and everlasting contribution was in the precedent he established.

The descriptions are brief, and it must be recalled that the actual wording is probably partly Geronimo Benivieni's. The post-mortem examinations were made with the definite purpose of determining the seat of disease or explaining symptoms referable to a given organ or part. The bodies were incised (*"incidere"*), not dissected (*"dissecare"*) as with Morgagni, and the results are of course correspondingly sketchy.

Some of the more interesting cases are worth recording:

No. 36: A relative by marriage vomited everything, being unable to retain food or medicine, gradually wasting away to skin and bone and finally dying. Benivieni opened his body "in the interest of the public good," and found an induration of the stomach reaching to the pylorus and preventing the passage of

ANTONII BENIVENII FLOREN, TINI MEDICI ET PHILOSOPHI DE ABDITIS NON NVLLIS AC MIRANDIS MORBORVM ET SA, NATIONVM CAVSIS .

De morbo quem uulgo Gallicuz uo, cant . Caput, Primum.

OVVM MORBI GENVS,
Anno Salutis nonagefimo fex,
to fupra mille qngentos a Chri
ftiana falute non folum Italiaz
fed fere totam Europá irrepfit.
Hoc ab Hifpania incipiens, per Italiam ip
fam primum, tum Galliam cæterasqz Euro
pæ prouincias late diffufuz mortales q plu
rimos occupauit . Incipiebant enim puftu
læ genere diuerfæ in genitalibus membris,
licet interduz fed rarenter in capite : & inde
per totum corpus diffúdebant̄ . Aliis qdez
plane minimeqz extantes : fed fcabræ tam̄
in fuperficie, & colore fubalbidæ : a quib9
fquamæ refoluebantur, & caro fub his cȯ
rofa apparebat . Aliis uaris fimiles figura
rotundæ : & ab his item fquamis leuiorib9
refolutis prominebat caro rubicundior :

A PAGE FROM ANTONIO BENIVIENI
Published in 1507

food. This was obviously an obstructive carcinoma of the pylorus.

No. 81: "Death from wind alone" (*"ex solo vento mors sub-sequuta"*). In this case everything was found normal, except that the viscera were full of gas. Dodoens half a century later concluded it was the intestines that were dilated with gas, i.e., the condition of tympany. The case was probably one of paralytic ileus, but whether due to an unrecognized peritonitis, or a mesenteric thrombosis or other cause, it is impossible to tell at this distance of four centuries.

No. 83: A robber who had been hanged on a gibbet was cut down and resuscitated. He returned to crime, was recaptured and this time more effectually hanged. "Marvelling at the wickedness of the man," says Benivieni, "they (his associates) went to great pains to secure a necropsy," and were surprised to find a "heart stuffed with hair" (*"cor pilis refertum"*). A case previously recorded in medical literature led Benivieni and his friends to believe this condition not only correlated with great wickedness but likewise "a sign of rare fortitude." We must not forget that these men lived in an age when anything seemed possible. The case was possibly one of simple fibrinous pericarditis, and there must have been associated lesions which Benivieni's friends, who apparently made the examination, overlooked.

No. 93: "A noble woman, Diamantes by name, recently passed away, prostrated by the pain of calculi." But it was no common case of gallstones, a condition with which Benivieni was quite familiar. In this case "these were not in the gall bladder as might be expected, except for one of black color and the size of a large dry chestnut, which was retained in its tunic; the rest were all in the panniculus, which was adherent to the liver, hanging from which they formed a sac." This was good observation, not difficult to be sure, but accurate as far as it went. Significant is the "as might be expected," showing Benivieni's thorough familiarity with ordinary cholelithiasis.

One of the most illuminating references is in an obscure case of intestinal obstruction in which the relatives refused necropsy, to Benivieni's great dejection (*"Sed nescio qua superstitione versi negantibus cognatis"*). Evidently he usually had more success in persuading the relatives of the deceased of the value of clearing up the case.

Not all of the descriptions are clear, e.g., the case of "callus among and obstructing the mesenteric veins." Possibly he was dealing with the enlarged lymph nodes of tuberculosis or typhoid fever. This is more likely than the usual interpretation of mesenteric thrombosis, a rarer condition. The ancient Greeks whom Benivieni followed, were apt to consider enlarged lymph nodes or tubercles (phymata) as coagulated humors obstructing the veins (See Galen, Chapter II).

He must often have overlooked the essential lesions, seizing upon what was readily apparent to the eye. In a number he mistook post-mortem changes for pathological lesions. He noted with care the "polyps" of the heart, as did all subsequent pathologists for nearly three centuries. These were of course simple post-mortem blood clots. We cannot delay with him too long, but should note that he left good descriptions of abscess of the hip joint, possibly tuberculous, of senile dry gangrene of the legs in several old gentlemen of Florence, "that black ulcer which the Greeks call gangrene," of hernias of several kinds, of fistulas, including vesico-rectal, of caries of the ribs, of ulcer of the jaw secondary to a carious tooth, of cicatrix following a burn, of twins of the Siamese type, and many other lesions of surgical interest. He was a good operator, and surgeons find his book as interesting historically as do pathologists. To be sure his explanations of what he saw were based entirely on the old humoral pathology. But he took the great step forward of searching out, as well as he could, the organic seat of the disease.

A younger contemporary of Benivieni, a pupil according to Puccinotti, was Alessandro Benedetti (about 1460-1525), professor of anatomy and one of the founders of the illustrious anatomical theater of Padua, to be graced later by Vesalius, Colombo, Fabricius of Aquapendente, the student Harvey and Morgagni. While military surgeon in Crete, Benedetti wrote a book full of original observations, recording among other pathological findings gallstones and malposition of the heart. Benedetti was held in the highest respect by medical writers of succeeding generations, and must be ranked with Benivieni in the impetus he gave to the pathologic-anatomical point of view. He is notable also for keen observations on the transmission of the virus of plague and the contagion of syphilis.

A little later than Benivieni we meet the robust figure of Berengario da Carpi (1470-1550), professor of surgery at Bologna, who boasts of the dissection of more than a hundred bodies. Some of these, according to Allbutt, may have been the bodies of pigs, but certainly Berengario dissected the human frame also, and most enthusiastically. His commentary on Mondino is a great text of pre-Vesalian anatomy, with the especial merit of illustrations. He mentions among other abnormalities a dilated heart. Berengario was a good friend of Benvenuto Cellini, who records in his frank way that da Carpi was "a surgeon of highest renown" who "in the course of other practice undertook the most desperate cases of the so-called French disease," for big fees to be sure, "an illness partial to priests, especially the richest of them." But after he left Rome, adds the truthful Cellini, "all the patients he had treated grew so ill that they were a hundred times worse off than before he came. He would certainly have been murdered if he had stopped." But the wise Berengario continued on his way, emphasizing anatomy, and promoting by his example, as Rayer says, if not by his results, the cause of its pathological branch.

Of the same period is the versatile Girolamo Fracastoro, physician, poet, cosmographer and natural philosopher. He is notable in pathology for his remarkable book on Contagion *(De Contagione et Contagiosis Morbis et Curatione)*, and his extended consideration of syphilis. The first defined contagion and contagious diseases clearly, committing the author to the contagious nature of two great plagues, typhus fever and consumption. Fracastoro drew a remarkable analogy between infection (he spoke of a transmissible *"virus"*) and the fermentation of wine, anticipating Pasteur by several centuries.

Fracastoro was a good deal of an astrologer, however, and, incredible as it may seem, was at first willing to assign the cause of the obviously contagious syphilis partly to the malign influence of the planets, particularly Mars and Saturn. Syphilis was at this time a fast augmenting pestilence, and in the easy manners of the time, its venereal transmission was for a time if not overlooked at least uncertain. It was commonly supposed to have originated in Spain with the return of Columbus' sailors from America, and its later virulent outbreak in Italy was attributed to the siege of Spanish Naples, once a possession of the house of Aragon, by Charles VIII of France, whose army contained Spanish mercenaries. The French called this new malady the "Neapolitan disease" and the Neapolitans retaliated with the more enduring *"Morbus Gallicus."* Fracastoro introduced the term "syphilis" in his celebrated poem *Syphilis sive Morbus Gallicus,* Syphilis being the name of the fictitious hero, who was afflicted with the disease for blaspheming the Sun-God. In a more serious prose study published in 1546, sixteen years after his famous poem, Fracastoro definitely emphasized its venereal origin, and gave an excellent account of its clinical course from the initial genital lesion to the late lesions in the mouth, pharynx and bones. Nicholas Massa of Venice, in 1532, had already described gummas in the dead body, calling them *"materiae albae viscosae."*

Fracastoro, like Benivieni and many other prominent physicians, speculated at length on the origin of syphilis, without settling the matter, and it is worth noting in passing that the problem is just as little settled today. It was well known in 1495. In addition to the Naples epidemic, which Sudhoff thinks may not have been syphilis at all, there was one in the same year in Barcelona. Ruy Díaz de Isla, in a work written about 1510, but not published for many years, was perhaps the first to suggest the American origin. He claimed he treated the sailors of Columbus for the disease on their return from Haiti in 1493. The great historians of the New World, Oviedo and Las Casas, both supported the view of American origin.

On the other hand many medical historians believe they have caught references to syphilis in medical literature prior to 1495. And Dodoens in the middle of the sixteenth century insisted that William of Saliceto (1270), Bernard Gordonius (fourteenth century) and Valescus of Taranta (1418) all described it. Whatever the origin, it certainly reached sudden epidemic proportions in the closing years of the fifteenth century, and in less than a hundred years extended to the confines of the civilized world. The extraordinary dissimilarity of its various lesions made a difficult problem for pathology, not entirely settled before the twentieth century. In its solution such notable figures as Fernel, Paré, Paracelsus, Lancisi, Morgagni, John Hunter and Virchow all played a part.

The sixteenth century has often been called the century of anatomy. What is generally unappreciated is that it was only slightly less a century of pathological anatomy. With dissection becoming commonplace in universities all over Europe, it was inevitable that observations of the ·abnormal should steadily accumulate.

Vesalius (1514-1564), Colombo (1516?-1559), Fallopius (1523-1562) and Eustachius (1524-1574) all made observations in pathology. Vesalius was familiar with aortic aneurysm (the earliest descriptions of which are credited to Antoine Saporta of Montpellier [died 1573]), and in 1555, in the case of a nobleman in Augsburg, diagnosed the condition during life. His diagnosis was confirmed two years later by necropsy, which was performed by

Augsburg physicians. Vesalius also made a number of judicial necropsies. According to Schenck von Grafenberg he intended to publish his pathological observations as a separate volume, and perhaps did put them in manuscript form. If so, they were probably lost in that temperamental outburst in which he burned many of his manuscripts before going to Spain. On the chance that it might have survived, a search for the manuscript was made by the French Ambassador at Madrid in 1812, without success. Vesalius' follower, Eustachius, in his gouty senescence, lamented, while recording a note on diseased kidneys, that he had not made a particular study of pathological anatomy rather than normal anatomy in his healthy and vigorous youth.

To be sure, much of the public dissection was of executed criminals, for the most part cut off in the prime of life, in normal health. Not much enrichment of pathological anatomy could be expected from such a source, although occasional surprises might be encountered, as in Benivieni's case (No. 83). It must not be forgotten, however, that dissection not infrequently followed a clandestine disinterment, after death from "natural causes," i.e., from disease, with pathological anatomy there to be observed, if the dissector were acute enough to recognize it. Finally there were such necropsies as Benivieni's, where the clinical data of the last illness were known. The Florentine's ready success in obtaining permission to make post-mortem examinations, secured by request exactly as today, shows that post-mortem study by reputable physicians was not regarded by the lay population as blasphemous. As a matter of fact when the occasion demanded, the bodies of dignitaries of the Church themselves were subjected to post-mortem examination. In 1410 Pietro d'Argellata examined the body of Pope Alexander V, who died suddenly and mysteriously in Bologna, and afterwards left a description of it in his *Surgery*.

Altogether a considerable body of information was gathering on the organic changes induced by disease, substantiating the beliefs of Galen and supplementing the observations of the surgeons. The first to codify this new knowledge was one of the greatest medical figures of the sixteenth century, Jean Fernel of Amiens (1497?-1558). Nothing serves better to illustrate the progress made in the first half of this century, than a comparison of the chief works of Benivieni and Fernel. Where the former was a brave pioneer groping his way in the dark, Fernel was a full-fledged pathologist.

This remarkable man was born in Picardy in 1497. His early

inclinations were toward philosophy and ancient languages, and for a time he devoted himself especially to mathematics, a training which, as Garrison says, doubtless had much to do with his later tendency to logical classification. Simultaneously he studied medicine, becoming doctor in 1530 and professor of medicine in the Paris faculty in 1534. His ability soon brought him an extensive practice, including notable members of the French court. He was physician to Diane de Poitiers, mistress of the dauphin, and after the latter's accession as Henry II, he attended both the king and his wife, the famous Catherine de Médicis, accompanying the royal pair on all their travels.

Fernel's zeal and industry in collecting the medical knowledge of his Greek and Arabian predecessors in the midst of a heavy practice was such that his health suffered. He has sometimes been called the French Galen, and yet is often cited as one of the first who attempted to throw off the yoke of Galen. He came too early in medical history to break with the teaching of humors, temperaments, and vital spirits of the ancients; yet he developed a more rational general pathology than they, and wrote a special pathology which in its organization fell little short of being modern. His famous *Medicina* (1554), in three parts, physiology, pathology, and therapeutics, became standard throughout Europe.

He classified diseases as general and special, the former including those of undetermined localization (*"morbi incertae sedis"*), and the latter those localized in an organ or part. Fevers fell in the first group, and were in turn classified as simple, putrid and pestilential. The special diseases were for purposes of systematization divided into three groups: (1) those affecting the parts above the diaphragm; (2) those involving the parts below; and (3) external diseases. As a sub-classification he distinguished (1) simple disease, affecting part of an organ; (2) compound, involving entire organs; and (3) complicated, in which the normal relations between parts were disturbed.

He distinguished, as we do today, symptoms and signs. Abnormalities in the pulse and urinary secretion ranked prominently in the latter group. This was a day when sober quacks of ponderous mien solemnly diagnosed everything from disappointed love to measles by naked-eye examination of a flask of the sufferer's urine. Fernel, the mathematician, wrote a chapter on *"urinae copia et paucitas, quid indicet,"* which would appeal to the most modern for its emphasis on the significance of quantitative variation in urinary output. He noted the reciprocal relation of urine and sweat, and the effect of obstruction in the urinary passages by tumors and calculi.

In the last three books of his *Pathologiae Libri VII* (1554)—the first medical work to be called a text of *Pathology*—he compiled succinctly the best knowledge of the time on organic abnormality in disease. Only enough to indicate his organization can be mentioned here. Discussing diseases of the head he recognized compression of the medulla or spinal cord as a possible cause of paralysis, although giving a fanciful humoral explanation also. He spoke of cavity (*"vomica"*) of the lung and abscess as identical, possibly confusing tuberculous and suppurative processes. In one of Fernel's *Consilia,* however, is a short necropsy protocol clearly describing an ordinary case of chronic ulcerative tuberculosis.

Cancer of the stomach is designated "abscess," in Fernel's time still the generic term for swelling, and ulceration of the tumor is mentioned, together with ulceration of the stomach from caustics. His consideration of diseases of parts below the diaphragm takes up in order: the stomach, the liver, the gall bladder, the spleen, the mesentery and "what they call the pancreas," the intestines, the kidneys, the uterus and the other generative organs. The last chapter discusses the *lues venerea,* on which Fernel was well informed, as indeed one must have been who practiced medicine in the promiscuous French court. He distinguished four types, with a suggestion of our modern four stages.

There is at times a certain stereotyping of description, suggesting assumption of a particular condition rather than its actual observation. In the case of both liver and kidney he lists as the usual abnormalities, "obstruction, scirrhous inflammation, abscess and ulcer." He was certainly familiar with obstruction of the outlet by calculus in each case, and his scirrhous inflammation of the liver probably included cirrhosis, as we may judge from its description as *"praeter naturam durus."* Yet he does not seem to have paid much attention to the somewhat analogous condition of the kidneys, which, although noticed from time to time, seems to have escaped the serious scrutiny of pathologists until the time of Richard Bright. According to Fernel, "inflammation properly considered nephritis is rare," a view probably taken directly from Galen. His treatment of abnormalities in the uterus, which had the benefit of surgical and obstetrical as well as post-mortem knowledge, is more nearly exhaustive.

In the pages on pathology in the *Medicina* he described what

PLATE V

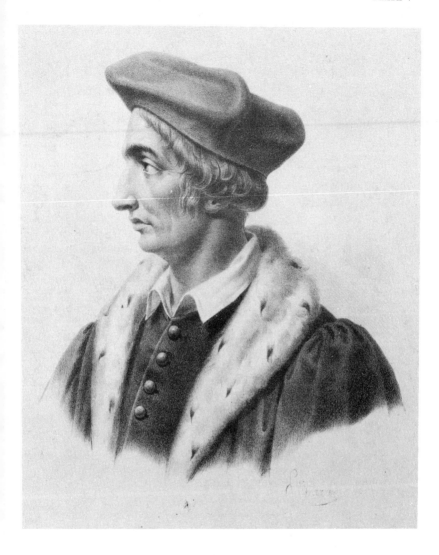

JEAN FERNEL (1497?-1558)

PLATE VI

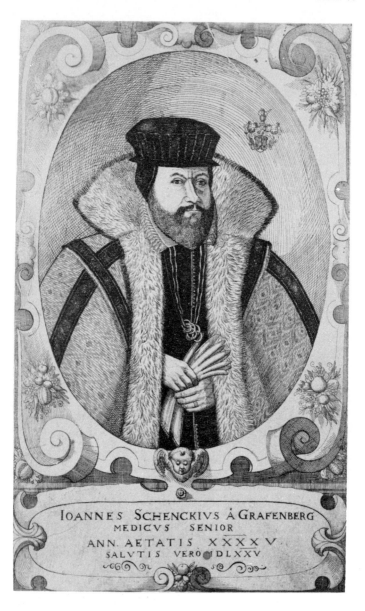

JOHANN SCHENCK VON GRAFENBERG (1530-1598)

was unquestionably appendicitis in a girl nine years old, with post-mortem examination, the only clear case of this disease on record until Heister's in 1711. He was an early student of aneurysms, and one of the first to suggest the syphilitic origin of some of them. He was a thorough Galenic humoralist on cancer, but knew of its frequent internal localization. He spoke of superficial growths of nodular character as sarcoma (*"sarcoma carius"*), including such diverse lesions as the chronic granulation tissue of healing ulcers, nasal polyps, and that jaw tumor known as epulis. The term sarcoma for centuries was used very loosely.

Altogether he had an extensive knowledge of pathological anatomy, and while he rambled vaguely about poisoning of the vital spirits, or assigned the cause of disease to the humors in a way that seems bizarre today, he located disease in the solid parts, and gave a great impetus to exact anatomical observation. In his systematization he was far ahead of his period. His *Pathology* was as suitable a text for teaching in his time as Matthew Baillie's, more than two hundred years later. He towered in this respect above his contemporaries and immediate followers, most of whom were content to assemble observations without systematizing them.

The most important competing classification was that of the Basel anatomist Felix Plater (1536-1614), who in fifty years dissected more than three hundred bodies, making numerous observations of pathologic-anatomical value. Plater, a practicing physician also, made a classification on the basis of symptoms. His pathological observations include sublingual calculi, giantism (he possessed the skeleton of a man nine feet tall), brain tumor, enlarged thymus in an infant, intestinal parasites, and cystic liver and kidneys associated with terminal anasarca. Plater is much quoted by all the latter compilers.

An enthusiast in the cause of pathological anatomy in the same century was Volcher Coiter of Groningen and Nuremberg (1534 to about 1590), a pupil of Fallopius and an excellent anatomist himself. He urged repeatedly that the authorities support with all their power the policy of post-mortem examination of persons dying of severe or puzzling disease. So imbued was he with the importance of pathologic-anatomical study that he gave up private practice for a position in military medicine, which afforded him more scope in this field. He is particularly noteworthy in pathology for his descriptions of cerebral and spinal meningitis.

An Italian contemporary, Marcello Donato of Mantua (second half of the sixteenth century) was equally forceful in his advocation of necropsy. His serious exhortation in his *De Medicina Historia Mirabili* (Mantua, 1586) is worth repeating in its entirety for its plain statement of the pathologist's two lasting problems: "Let those who interdict the opening of bodies well understand their errors. When the cause of a disease is obscure, in opposing the dissection of a corpse which must soon become the food of worms, they do no good to the inanimate mass, and they cause a grave damage to the rest of mankind; for they prevent the physicians from acquiring a knowledge which may afford the means of great relief eventually to individuals attacked by a similar disease. No less blame is applicable to those physicians who, from laziness or repugnance, love better to remain in the darkness of ignorance than to scrutinize laboriously the truth, not reflecting that by such conduct they render themselves culpable toward God, themselves and society at large." (From Renouard's *History of Medicine,* Comiegnys' translation.)

The book is chiefly a collection of the unusual observations of others, including Benivieni, Vesalius, Colombo, Dodoens and others less notable. Such compilations were soon to become very common. Donato spent eleven years in getting this together and showed an extraordinary indulgence toward such unlikely stories as the sweating of blood and the passage of a kernel of wheat through the ureter. Nevertheless he included some valuable records. Among them is the first good pathologic-anatomical description of a carcinoma of the rectum. This occurred in an old man, who was severely constipated, and whose rectum was not permeable to a wax candle. The necropsy disclosed in the upper part of the rectum, which was severely contracted, an elevated, gland-like tumor.

We have seen how the new science of pathological anatomy was being cultivated in Italy, France, Switzerland and Germany. The Netherlands added a share in the persons of Rembert Dodoens and Pieter van Foreest. The former is perhaps best known for his contributions to botany, the professorship of which he held at Leyden. In those days, particularly in the Netherlands (see Ruysch, later), the chairs of botany and anatomy were frequently combined, and the incumbent practiced medicine.

Dodoens (1517-1585), who studied originally in Louvain and traveled extensively in France, Italy and Germany, coming into contact with the most celebrated physicians of the time, thoroughly appreciated the gain from post-mortem examination in the understanding of disease. In the dedication of his *Medicinalium Observationum Exempla Rara* he notes that this advantage was denied to Hippocrates and Galen, and adds, "It is the greater privilege of a later age to open human bodies and by this means study concealed affections and their hidden causes." This book, like that of Donato, is a collection of rarities, but from Dodoens' own practice. Fifty-four cases are described, relatively few of them of outstanding importance.

The chief merit is the method of report, notable for its careful distinction between the subjective and objective. In only a few of the fifty-four cases is a necropsy recorded, but when it is present, the method of case report is always as follows: (1) clinical history, (2) necropsy, in strictly objective terms, and (3) the scholion, or Dodoens' subjective interpretation of the case, along with citations of literature or any other matter appearing to him as relevant.

Among the cases recorded are: hydrophobia thirty-seven years after a dogbite (no post-mortem); tonsillar abscess; fibrinous bronchitis with expectoration of bronchial casts and death ultimately from pulmonary hemorrhage (no post-mortem); gangrene of the lung (or pulmonary infarction, in the opinion of Meerbeck; necropsy performed); gastric ulcer in a woman sixty years old, who had suffered from epigastric pain for years (necropsy performed, but not clear, as the ulcers are described as on the outside of the stomach and on the neighboring organs); and a complicated case, with gangrene of one foot, cachexia and apparently terminal peritonitis, possibly secondary to a malignant tumor (necropsy performed, but the report too brief for positive interpretation). Dodoens, of course, explained these lesions of the solid parts in humoral terms. Apoplexy, for example, resulted from sudden obstruction of the cerebral ventricles by crude, pituitous or phlegmatic humors, often mixed with blood. We see a trace here the confusion that existed from the time of the ancients up to Wepfer, between cerebral hemorrhage and meningitis, expressed somewhat vaguely in their distinction between sanguinous and serous apoplexy.

Pieter van Foreest (1522-1597) of Delft, sometimes called the Dutch Hippocrates, was unusual for his time in that he was less interested in the rarities than the common phenomena of morbid states. He published records of about a thousand cases, with some attention to morbid anatomy, but a not altogether successful correlation with physiological disturbance.

The greatest of the compilers of this period was Johann Schenck von Grafenberg, (1530-1598). He studied chiefly in the old university town of Tübingen, practiced for a time in Strassburg and utimately settled in Freiburg as city physician, where he died in 1598. In the closing years of his life (1584-97), he brought out his great *Observationum Medicarum Rararum . . . Libri VII,* which was reprinted several times before 1665. In it are collected the observations of a lifetime of medical reading, to which are added a number from his own wide experience and that of relatives and friends in medical practice. A great many of the citations are concise summaries of post-mortem discoveries. Clarity of author reference and good indexing are conspicuous merits of the book.

The folio, which runs to 900 pages, opens with the usual laudatory good wishes of distinguished medical contemporaries. Of especial significance, however, in the introduction, as illustrating Schenck's point of view, is a series of quotations on the educational benefit derived from examining dead bodies in obscure disease, taken from Galen, Pliny, Alessandro Benedetti, Johann Kentmann (a physician and mineralogist [1518-1574], who was much interested in calcareous deposits of all sorts in the body), Volcher Coiter and Marcello Donato. The organization of the text is the usual one, followed by the later compilers like Bonet, on the basis of symptoms referable to an anatomical part, beginning with the head.

Schenck's book is the easiest present source for the numerous pathological observations of Sylvius, Vesalius, and Colombo, which are scattered widely in their own more strictly anatomical works. Probably few medical authors of note from the time of Hippocrates are overlooked. Avenzoar's *"verruca ventriculi"* is noted. Bauhin's observation of blood gushing forth on opening the head of a man who died from apoplexy, and Garnerus' finding in a dissection of 1578 of a spleen weighing 23 pounds and a liver weighing 11 pounds, most probably a case of splenomyelogenous leukemia, may be cited as examples of the range of pathological discovery quoted. Schenck's own records concerning intestinal parasites are particularly good. On the whole, the work, while very far from a modern text of pathology, is a remarkable collection of observations preserved in a form permitting recognition in the light of modern knowledge.

Naturally the surgeons, with their unique opportunity for the study of pathological changes in the living body, made numerous contributions to the growing science. The foremost of these, the sturdy Ambroise Paré, (1510-1590), did much to advance pathology through anatomy by popularizing Vesalius in common French in an introductory compendium to his *Surgery*. Paré, who came up from the ranks of the barber surgeons, and was unable to write a Latin thesis for his admission to the college of St. Côme, was one of the first to dare the use of his native tongue in scientific publication. For the first time we hear of *"tumeurs contre nature"* instead of the time honored *"tumores praeter naturam."* He was not a whit past Galen in his explanation of these, but he left some excellent descriptions, showing familiarity with internal cancer, and with him we see a growing conception of the phenomenon of metastasis, in his emphasis on the swelling of the axillary lymph nodes in cancer of the breast. The story of his first omission of the irritant boiling oil in the treatment of gun-shot wounds, and foreshadowing of asepsis, is too familiar to warrant repetition. Paré was well acquainted with aneurysms, not only those due to violence, but also the internal kind, and like Fernel considered syphilis a predisposing cause.

His Teutonic contemporary, Wilhelm Fabry of Hilden, (Fabricius Hildanus, 1560-1634), sometimes called the Ambroise Paré of Germany, also attached great importance to pathological anatomy. He was an excellent student of normal anatomy (even recommending its cultivation by priests and lawyers that they might apply torture with more effect and discretion to criminals), and left good records, with drawings, of congenital departures from the normal. He made a notable collection of bones showing the healing of fractures. But his chief contributions to pathology were his treatise on burns, distinguishing the classical three degrees, and his great work on *Gangrene, Hot and Cold,* which was published in 1593 and went through eleven editions. He was, unfortunately, firmly attached to the almost universal practice of deliberately inducing suppuration in wounds by the use of all sorts of irritants, the value of which he explained as usual on the ground that the process afforded an outlet for the "vicious humors."

Altogether the sixteenth century enormously advanced men's knowledge on location of disease in the solid parts. The theory of original cause lagged, however, just as it does today. Few had the courage to depart much from the confident assertions of Galen, whose humoral and vitalistic-spirit pathology still reigned supreme. The few daring innovators, like Paracelsus, who publicly burned Galen's works, together with Avicenna's, at Basel in 1527, for the most part only substituted a still less tangible general pathology. Paracelsus (1493-1541), the great swashbuckler of the medical Renaissance, quarrelsome but intellectually independent, an alchemist by training, classified etiology in disease on a mystical, vitalistic basis with a series of governing *"entia,"* but foreshadowed modern chemical pathology in his conception of precipitation in the formation of calculi and gouty deposits, and was the first to correlate cretinism and endemic goiter.

His follower, the Belgian mystic, van Helmont (1577-1644), another forerunner of modern biological chemistry, developed a physiological and pathological system that seems outlandish to us; but he had the courage of his convictions, and practiced what he preached. As John Lobkowiz says, "Helmont was pious, learned and famous, a sworn enemy to Galen and Aristotle. The sick never languished long under his care, being always killed or cured in two or three days." In his own serious illness of 1640, van Helmont saved himself, if we may trust his own statement, by taking in succession shavings from the genital organs of a stag, a dram of goat's blood, and urine boiled with crab's eyes, a nicety of pharmacological combination almost surpassing the Arabians.

Van Helmont lived into the time of William Harvey, but took no advantage of the *De Motu Cordis et Sanguinis.* In his physiology, life was regulated by a head *Archaeus* seated in the stomach and spleen, and a number of minor *archaei* in other organs, with digestive ferments, van Helmont's own discovery, under their control. The emotional outbursts of the Archaeus, upsetting the normal distribution of ferments, were responsible for disease. If a woman's breast were injured, the Archaeus, furious at the insult, produced a tumor. The mythical Archaeus was thus substituted for the *atra bilis,* but we must not forget that van Helmont clearly distinguished cancer from other lesions, and that in the field of ferments, which lay back of his conception of the Archaeus, he was a great experimenter, and laid part of the foundation of modern physiology. Inasmuch as knowledge of autolysis or self digestion of tissue underlies our modern understanding of the degenerative changes in pathological lesions, we must accord van Helmont an honorable place in the development of chemical pathology.

On the whole, however, the balance of power remained with Galen, in spite of Vesalius and the anatomical pathologists. As a matter of fact, Vesalius, as well as the rest, supported Galen so frequently that in some fields the Pergamene's hold on general pathology was even tightened. The break-up began only with Harvey.

CHAPTER IV

The Seventeenth Century

With the sixteenth century anatomy was revolutionized, and a sound basis laid for the accurate recognition of morbid change. Necropsies for the purpose of detecting this change, as well as routine dissections, had become common. A new thing on the face of the earth, printing with movable type, had made the new anatomical knowledge available to all who could read. The records were at first widely scattered, and buried in unrelated material. A group of compilers soon arose, however, who collected the post-mortem examinations of others, usually to supplement their own. Their attention was taken for the most part, unfortunately, by the curiosities and rarities, from which no comprehensive science of pathological anatomy could be constructed. A few had the good sense to hold fast to the commonplace and therefore important, however, and one brilliant physician among them, Jean Fernel, codified the first text of *Pathology* as part of a *System of Medicine*. Etiology and pathogenesis, nevertheless, remained in the control of Galenic and Arabian thought.

In the seventeenth century, that bewildering period when science and literature flourished with incredible vigor in the face of religious strife, the Thirty Years' War and the English Revolution, came William Harvey's (1578-1657) *De Motu Cordis et Sanguinis* (1628), a work of incalculable influence on general pathology. To appreciate its significance we must recall that as long as men remained ignorant of the circulation of the blood, believing in a simple ebb and flow of arterial and venous systems, those great phenomena of fatal hemorrhage, passive hyperemia, edema and general anasarca, embolism, infarction, pyemia, miliary tuberculosis, neoplastic growth, and all the evils that follow in their train, could only remain unrecognized or incomprehensible. Probably no single discovery has been of more far-reaching effect in pathology.

Harvey's service to the growing science of pathology was not limited to his discovery of the circulation. He made special contributions in the same field. He left a good description of a heart hypertrophy, apparently the result of an incompetent aortic valve, for the aorta is described as greatly widened, and sketched the symptoms which preceded death in this case. He also described a ruptured heart, with a finger-wide tear in the left ventricle.

During his Physicianship in Ordinary to Charles I, at the king's command he made a post-mortem examination of the body of Thomas Parr, who died at the reputed age of 152 years. Harvey was cautious in committing himself on the actual cause of death, but expressed the opinion that Parr would have lived longer had he paid the same attention to his diet after coming to London as before. Unfortunately he does not tell us what sort of diet enabled Parr to live as long as he did.

In the sixteenth century printing came to the aid of the newly developing pathology. In the seventeenth we see for the first time, nearly a century after the publication of Jan Calcar's beautiful plates in Vesalius' *Fabrica,* illustrations of pathological lesions. One of the first to supplement his descriptions in this way was the surgeon Marco Aurelio Severino (1580-1656), a product of the late school of Salerno, who lived long in Naples, where he was professor of anatomy, and finally died there of the plague. He is sometimes considered the reformer of surgery in Italy, and his great book *De Recondita Abscessuum Natura* (1632) may fitly be considered the first text of surgical pathology.

It is a complete treatise on swellings, which is still all the word "abscess" conveyed. If any particular swelling was left out, it was that which we call abscess today. His tumor pathology is perhaps his best. He described tumors of the genital organs in both sexes, and colossal neoplasms, presumably sarcomas, of bones. He classified breast tumors in four groups, and his *Mammarum strumae ("per quae differant a scirrhis")* is one of the best early discussions of malignancy and benignity in tumors of this organ.

Like all writers of his time, he wrote voluminously on syphilis, quoting Benedetti, Fernel and Laurent Joubertus on internal syphilis. He speaks himself of ulceration of the esophagus and trachea, and pustules of the lung and liver, and describes a cadaver he dissected in Naples in which the disease had ex-

PLATE VII

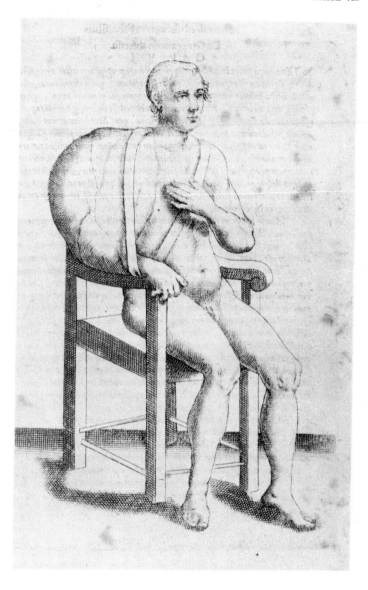

TUMOR OF THE HUMERUS
From the *De Recondita Abscessuum Natura* of Marco
Aurelio Severino, 1632

PLATE VIII

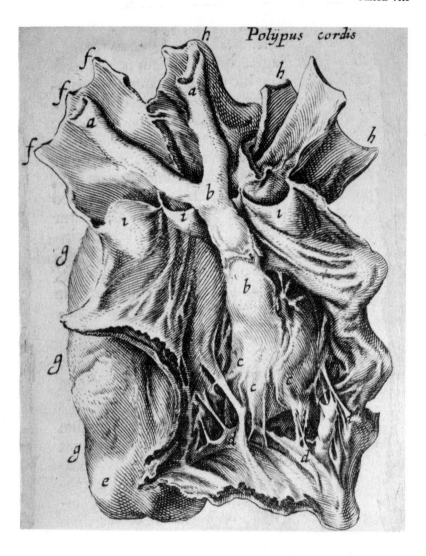

"POLYP" OF THE HEART
From the *Observationes Medicae* of Nicolaes Tulp, 1641

tended from the original lesion, destroying the left vas deferens
and internal glands, and forming a large ulcerating bubo. This
was probably gonorrhoea or chancroid and not syphilis. Nor is it
likely that the other ulcerations and pustules were syphilitic.
There is little doubt that many of the early descriptions of the
lues venerea were not descriptions of syphilis at all, and that the
mistaken diagnoses of a period only too willing to believe the

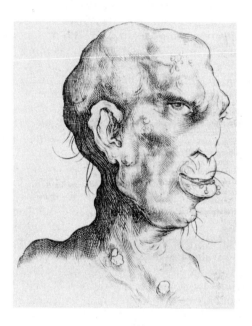

HEAD ILLUSTRATING DISCUSSION OF SYPHILIS
In Marco Aurelio Severino's *De Recondita Abscessuum
Natura* 1632

worst of the new plague, are responsible for a much exaggerated
notion of its early virulence.

With the final bloody repudiation of Spanish authority and
rise of the Dutch republic, the great Dutch schools of medicine,
already notable, became still more productive in the seventeenth
century. Nicolaes Tulp of Amsterdam (1593-1674) was one of the
first to profit by the new freedom. This celebrated man, familiar

as the central figure in Rembrandt's *School of Anatomy*, was a pupil of Pieter Pauw and later professor of anatomy. He was, moreover, a popular physician, with the distinction of being the first doctor in democratic Amsterdam to use a carriage in visiting his patients. He also stood high in civic affairs, being several times burgomaster. His political influence is believed to have been exerted in favor of scientific advance in the medical school. He is known in anatomy for his discovery of the ileocaecal valve (shared with Bauhin) and his excellent description of the lacteals. He also brought out the first Amsterdam pharmacopeia.

His contributions to pathology are no less notable. He was much interested in cancer and calculi. Among his numerous notes on malignant tumors is the first clear description of carcinoma of the bladder. A bladder-intestinal fistula was diagnosed in life from the fact that the patient passed urine by rectum, and post-mortem examination disclosed a tumor of the bladder with perforation into the colon. He described several cases of carcinoma of the breast, which he believed contagious, citing the case of a servant girl who acquired such a cancer from attending her mistress long and faithfully for the same disease. He removed a sixteen-pound tumor, undoubtedly a sarcoma, from the femur of a young woman, but she died of recurrence. He recorded what was unquestionably a cancer of the esophagus, "a tumor-like carcinoma" with stricture, such that he could scarcely get a probe through it. And he gave a good description of a hydatidiform mole, "a shapeless, bloody, vesicular mass, coming away bit by bit, filling an entire bucket," sharing with another Amsterdam physician, Lamzweerde, the honor of first describing this type of tumor. Altogether he had wide experience in this branch of pathology.

Tulp's great work, his *Observationes Medicae* (1641), like Severino's, was illustrated. Among the woodcuts are: nasal polyps, the casts of fibrinous bronchitis (which like Galen he considered vascular products, *"integra vena a pulmone rejecta"*), an expectorated fragment of a gangrenous lung (good), tapeworms, renal and bladder calculi, spina bifida (excellent), congenitally united twins, umbilical fistula and what purports to be hydrops of a bicornuate uterus, but may be bilateral cystic ovary (the last two illustrated also on his title page).

His *Observationes* also include hydrocephalus, tumors of the eye, ulcer of the palate, wounds, fractures, beri-beri Indorum, (sharing with Bontius the first description), gangrene of the legs, without recognition of the cause, and the inescapable "polyp" of the heart. Tulp seems to have scented something wrong here, but figured the usual post-mortem artifact in his illustrations (see Plate VIII).

A still more commanding figure in Dutch medicine is Franciscus Sylvius, (Franz de le Boë, 1614-1672), born in Hanover, Germany, trained chiefly in Basel, and professor in Leyden from 1648 until his death. He is particularly noted in medicine for his founding of the iatrochemical school, and his teaching on the specific pathological anatomy of tuberculosis.

The basis of the iatrochemical medicine, which later numbered Willis and Boerhaave among its adherents, was a new kind of humoral pathology. Sylvius was well versed in the current inorganic chemistry, probably quite familiar with Glauber's discoveries on the nature of salts, convinced by Harvey's teaching, and much impressed by van Helmont's discoveries of body ferments. And on this substantial foundation he erected his physiology and doctrine of pathogenesis.

He believed, and quite correctly, that acid and alkaline elements were normally balanced in the circulating blood, but susceptible to the action of the ferments, which might disturb the balance. As we look back through nearly three centuries, we see that Sylvius had clearly grasped a concept that we are sometimes naïvely inclined to think modern, viz., that of acidosis and alkalosis, but he erred like so many of his age in attempting to build an all-embracing system on a doctrine of restricted application. He distinguished disease due to excess alkali on the one hand or excess acid on the other, in a way that bears no relation to modern ideas, and of course treated his patients according to his view of the chemical indications. His notions, too, on the nature of fermentation, to him practically equivalent to the effervescence from adding acid to a carbonate, were imaginary. Rayer says that he made observation the keynote of systems, without realizing that his own, less than any other, was founded on exact observance. In his own lifetime, however, his reputation and influence were enormous, and unquestionably his views, however erroneous, stimulated greatly the development of physiological chemistry.

Sylvius was no mere theorist. He opened a prodigious number of cadavers, and will always be remembered as the first to recognize clearly and unmistakably the relation of the tubercle to tuberculosis. The ancients had drawn good clinical pictures of the disease, and vaguely distinguished "phymata" as an accompanying abnormality. But no such thing as a constant and characteristic lesion was recognized before Sylvius. He saw tubercles in the lungs of consumptives and described their progression into cavities. Separating the wheat from the considerable chaff, it is possible to construct a good working pathological anatomy of tuberculosis from Sylvius' observations. Such a reorganization would, however, probably furnish a wrong impression, and detract from the greater merit of Laënnec in this field. One of Sylvius' great contributions was the recognition of tuberculosis of the lymph glands in the mediastinum, neck and mesentery. But he was confused and appears at times to have considered the tubercle itself a gland developing abnormally in a different sort of tissue. But there is shrewd and correct deduction in his statement that "even when these glands are extremely small in the mesentery and sides of the neck while they are in the natural state, they grow prodigiously in size and hardness in disease." He concluded that the same glands may be in the body normally, but too small to be detected.

As etiology, he adduced all the views of the ancients (see Galen, Chap. 2), but supplemented them with his own chemical humoral pathology of abnormal juices, a condition which he considered hereditary.

While Sylvius was building a new physiological doctrine and fitting it into a medical system, an equally influential figure, Thomas Bartholin of Copenhagen (1616-1680), was dominating the rapidly growing science of anatomy. Himself the son of a great anatomist and scholar, Kaspar Bartholin, and related to most of the prominent physicians of his country, many of them intimate at the Danish court, he received a most careful, scholarly training. For nine years he studied and taught philosophy, ethics, theology, mathematics and finally medicine in Leyden, Paris, Montpellier, Padua and Basel. While in Leyden he brought out a new edition of his father's *Anatomy*, which was translated into several languages, including the Chinese, and from which the physicians of Europe learned their anatomy for fifty years.

He ultimately returned to Copenhagen, where he took the chair of anatomy, one of the three chief professorships of the medical faculty. He was extremely popular. His audiences included the king himself. His most important direct contribution to the subject was on the lymphatics. But teaching was not to his liking and in 1656 he retired to his country manor at Hagestedgaard, retaining, however, his academic and certain judicial connections, to devote himself to writing and correspondence for the rest of his life. Out of this scholarly retirement came his *Acta Medica Philosophica* (1673-80), a series of treatises by a number of eminent men of science under Bartholin's editorship, practically constituting a medical periodical, and one of the first in the world. Reprinted and translated, these had a wide distribution. He also published several volumes of personal correspondence with scientific men.

Bartholin thus did much to establish that intercourse of publication which is essential to scientific progress. His genius for editing, and his own fluent pen, far more than his individual research, give him a permanent place in medicine. Personally he was an anachronism, an extensively read scholar of antiquity, uncritical and courteously credulous of the extraordinary and even the impossible. Sirens and horned women, men born from goats, and all sorts of human and animal curiosities share his pages on even terms with clear descriptions of abscess of the brain following skull fracture, tumors and other lesions of the pancreas with diabetes (polyuria), and excellent accounts of urinary calculi, which must have been far more common then than now.

Some of these observations came from the skillful prosectors he had brought to his own anatomical theater, and a few from his own hand. A greater number are his own personal records of necropsies seen while studying with Sylvius in Leyden, Vesling in Padua, Trullus in Rome, etc. In his quiet retreat at Hagestedgaard he had unlimited opportunity for correlating these scattered observations into a system. But his was not that type of mind. He repeated Pieter Pauw's (1564-1614) observation of "much yellow water filling the thorax and abdomen from dyscrasia of the ventricle of the heart," as an isolated observation of a curiosity, all unknowing that under his pen flowed the statement of a great truth in pathology.

Pathological anatomy was fast overhauling normal anatomy, and with this period comes the partial understanding of apoplexy, always a favorite source of speculation with the ancients. The credit for this discovery goes chiefly to Johann Jakob Wepfer of Schaffhausen (1620-1695), one of the most celebrated physicians of the seventeenth century, whose interest was attracted particularly to diseases of the head. Like Benivieni, in the fatal cases of his private practice he went to all lengths to secure permission for necropsy, and deeply regretted his failures, as for example in connection with a case of hydrocephalus, where

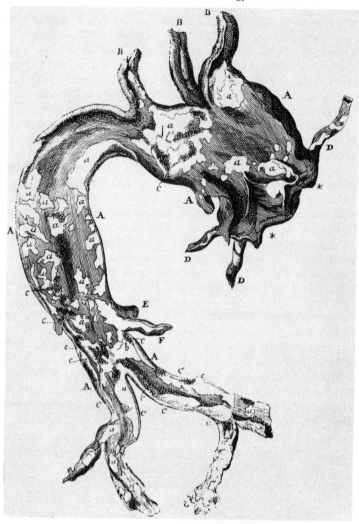

THE AORTA OF JOHANN JAKOB WEPFER (1620-1695)
Published in the posthumous edition of his book on
Diseases of the Head, 1727

neither prayer nor bribery availed (*"sed nec prece nec pretio
quicquam a defuncti uxore et affinibus impetrare valui"*).

Wepfer's most important discovery by far was the relation of
cerebral hemorrhage to certain types of apoplexy, and his de-

tection of the predisposing aneurysms of the small vessels. Brunner also described these little aneurysms shortly afterwards, but, as Morgagni says, "on this matter Wepfer is more clear." The clinical correlation with the lesions as revealed by post-mortem examination was excellent. Other good observations in his works concern tumors of the face and head, scrofula and syphilitic ulceration of the hard palate, occurring in a man with severe initial symptoms of syphilis six years previously.

Wepfer's own last illness illustrates well the medical acumen of the period. It is described by relatives in the *Memoria Wepferiana* prefacing a posthumous edition of his great book on the head, which records his life, travels, and positions as well as his final sickness, and concludes with a picture of the great man's aortic trunk from the semilunar valves to the femoral arteries (page 54). The case was clinically one of cardiac asthma (*"non nisi erectus respirare potuit"*), and it is particularly noteworthy that a necropsy was performed "as *customary*." This was on January 28, 1695. The Clarissimus Dr. D. Pfister officiated, "a most skilled doctor of medicine and surgery," making a careful and accurate post-mortem examination in which the condition of all organs was noted. The heart was recorded as enlarged, with a bony substance in its structure close to the pulmonic orifice. The aorta revealed what we now recognize as senile sclerosis, containing plaques of bony consistency particularly prominent and hard to cut in the neighborhood of the coeliac and renal arteries. This, let us note, was nearly three quarters of a century before the appearance of Morgagni's *Seats and Causes of Disease,* so often credited with the beginnings of pathological anatomy.

While such rapid strides were being made on the continent, anatomical knowledge of certain organs was being greatly advanced in England, particularly by Glisson and Willis. Francis Glisson of London (1597-1677), called by Boerhaave "the most accurate anatomist that ever lived," by his researches on the liver provided that anatomical basis indispensable for accurate knowledge of its pathology. He was also a good osteologist and gave one of the first clear descriptions of rickets. He is of still more importance to pathology for his recognition of irritability in tissues, a doctrine developed particularly by Haller.

Thomas Willis of London (1621-1675), whose name has been made immortal in the "Circle of Willis," likewise did not confine his scientific attention to normal anatomy. He was a great clinician, and an industrious investigator of the anatomical

lesions associated with disease. He was an extravagant humoralist, however, as regards its cause, with a leaning toward
the iatrochemical doctrines. A queer, rather ungraceful figure,
with admirers and almost abusive detractors, he has given rise to
much discussion on the originality of many of his observations.
He lived in a time of bitter strife, through which he remained a
staunch Royalist, taking great chances in the Cromwell regime.
His reward came with the Restoration in a professorship which
enabled him to pursue his scientific bent without molestation.

His observations of most importance in pathology are largely
in relation to the nervous system, to the normal anatomy of
which he had devoted himself diligently. He confirmed Wepfer on the hemorrhagic nature of apoplexy, and in his discussions on the cause of convulsions, on which he wrote special
treatises, are descriptions which may be interpreted as meningitis, although they are far from clear.

His work on phthisis is important, a disease to which he believed all chest ailments might lead "as small streams lead to
big lakes." He took exception of the current belief in "phthisis
as a wasting of the whole body from an ulceration of the lungs,"
noting that ulceration is not always present, and recording a
case in which there were "scattered through the lungs in every
part tubercles or stones of sandy matter," possibly a case of
chronic miliary tuberculosis.

He wrote a good treatise on scurvy, and his notations on
"epidemical dysentery" are interpreted as an early description
of typhoid fever. He states that some years it was worse than the
plague and due to "a certain infection impressed on the blood
and so intimately confused with it under the form of a vapor
or sincere humor that it cannot be pulled away; wherefore the
thrusting forward toward the intestine unlocks the little mouths
of the arteries and makes there little ulcers and exudations or
flowing forth of blood." A bit fanciful, but not unreasonable for
the seventeenth century. Willis always had a ready explanation
for any pathological lesion he saw, and his great *Practice of
Physick* has been described as not so much a book as a small
library, representing largely his own original, industrious research and ideas.

Another great work of the time on tuberculosis was the
Phthisiologia (1689) of Richard Morton (1635-1698). In spite of
its repetition and inconsistencies, and fantastic humoral explanations, it was clinically exhaustive for the period. From
his descriptions of phthisical lungs it is possible to interpret

caseo-nodular, ulcerative, and calcareo-caseous types of tuber-culosis, as well as caseous and ulcerative tuberculosis of the kidney, but on the whole little is added to the tuberculosis pathology of Sylvius.

The greatest English medical figure of the period was Thomas Sydenham (1624-1689), whose late acquisition of his doctorate in medicine (when he was 52) must afford much encouragement to medical students in this day of increasingly lengthy and ar-duous pre-graduation requirement. Sydenham took Hippocrates as his model, and was an example of gifted simplicity. He was a humoralist, without being a theorist. He recognized only ob-servation and practical experience, considering anatomy and physiology interesting of themselves, but not essential in the training of a medical practitioner. He conceived of disease quite simply as "a vigorous effort of nature to throw off morbific mat-ter and thus recover the patient." This emphasis on the healing power of nature was his greatest and lasting teaching, although he was an active therapeutist too, giving mercury in syphilis in enormous dosage and using herbs in profusion. He distinguished acuteness and chronicity in the speed and ease of removal of morbid material, wrote extensively on "inflammation of the blood," and considered unknown influences of the atmosphere important in the origin of disease, but did little toward real advance in the subject of pathology.

While the science was progressing as we have seen in the Netherlands, Denmark, Germany and England, in Italy the tra-dition of the brilliant anatomists of the Renaissance was being upheld. Popes and princes ardently supported anatomical and physiological studies, and pathological anatomy was beginning to be thought of as an independent discipline. In Rome, Gio-vanni Riva (1627-1677), physician to Pope Clement IX, a dis-tinguished anatomist and surgeon, established a special society for discussions of pathological anatomy, and founded a museum for pathological specimens in association with one of the hos-pitals. Riva made a number of important observations himself in pathology, particularly on aortic aneurysms.

The greatest figure of the century in Italian medicine is probably Marcello Malpighi (1628-1694), a graduate of Bologna, who began his teaching in Pisa in 1656. Distinguished in fields as widely separated as comparative anatomy and plant mor-phology, a convincing writer against the teaching of spontaneous generation, he is notable particularly for his discovery of the capillaries and red blood corpuscles and his masterly work on the minute structure of the kidneys, lungs, and spleen. He was thus one of the founders of histology, and shares the honor of introducing the microscope into medicine.

The invention of the compound microscope is a matter of some dispute, but the brothers Hans and Zacharias Janssen in Middelburg, Holland, are commonly credited with the manufacture of the first one, which is said to have been a foot and a half long. Cornelis Drebbel of Alkmaar, Holland, almost simultaneously made a better one, and to him the introduction of the instrument is really due. Another Dutchman, industrious beyond words, Antonj van Leeuwenhoek of Delft (1632-1723), accomplished its ultimate popularization, confirming Malpighi's discovery of the capillaries and blood corpuscles, and making extensive and important original observations on all sorts of subvisible forms of life. Previously, however, Athanasius Kircher of Fulda (1601-1680) studied putrefaction with the microscope and even attempted to find the cause of plague by examining the blood of plague patients. He took up where Fracastoro left off; Garrison calls him the first to state in explicit terms the doctrine of a *"contagium animatum"* as the cause of infectious disease. Jan Swammerdam of Amsterdam (1637-1680) and Robert Hooke of London (1635-1703) share with these men the great distinction of introducing into medicine this instrument of incalculable value.

Malpighi's contribution to pathology was not limited to the start he gave the indispensable sister science of histology. He made important gross observations, describing aortic sclerosis well in his report on his post-mortem examination of Cardinal Bonacairsi, and leaving descriptions of osteomyelitis and what was probably lymphogranulomatosis. He also made the usual mistake of his day, and wrote a tract *De polypo cordis*.

Malpighi died November 29, 1694, two months before Wepfer, of that apoplexy which Wepfer had described so well. Malpighi's necropsy, like Wepfer's, throws a good light on the post-mortem skill of those pre-Morgagnian days. It was performed by Baglivi in the presence of Lancisi, among others, who contributed the findings to the Royal Society of London, which had recently begun publishing its transactions. The heart was large and the left ventricle abnormally thick. There was no polypus. The right kidney was small, with dilated pelvis, and there was a stone in the bladder. The right ventricle of the brain contained two ounces of extravasated blood, and the left an ounce of "yellow phlegm."

The ascribed cause of the hemorrhage, however, shows the almost unbreakable hold of the ancient humoral pathology and the new humoralism of the iatrochemical school; for the revelations of the necropsy "proved that the conglobated glands in the whole body had thrown into the mass of blood an acid lymph, and that the conglomerated glands of the hypochondria, especially those of the liver, had thrown into it a melancholy humor, and that these two sorts of humor being carried into the vessels of the brain had disposed the blood to coagulate there, and that these having corroded and broken through the tunics which served for a stop to them, they had run into the cavities, where they caused death without a remedy" (Translation by W. G. MacCallum).

Giorgio Baglivi (1669-1707), Malpighi's pupil, and later professor in Rome, who made the examination, was nevertheless doing the best he could to break away from humoral pathogenesis. Like Glisson, he was impressed by 'the irritability of tissues, and inclined to seat disease in the solid parts without taking the humors into account. He has been considered the leading exponent of the Italian *iatro-physical* school, on account of his emphasis on the mechanics of physiology. He likened the body to a complicated piece of machinery with teeth like shears, a stomach like a flask, blood vessels for conducting tubes, and a pump, the heart.

He rejuvenated the old solidism of the methodists in ascribing disease to changes in the tone of the solid parts. His speculative general pathology has been called an "effusion of youth." Yet he was a careful prosector also and added specifically to the growing knowledge of pathological anatomy. Under the term *"Febris mesenterica"* he described the intestinal changes and mesenteric lymph node swelling characteristic of typhoid fever, making a considerable advance over Willis, if they were describing the same thing.

The end of the century witnessed a new crop of *specilegia* or assemblages of necropsy reports. The greatest, by far, of these is the *Sepulchretum sive Anatomia Practica* of Bonet (1679), a book especially notable in the history of pathology because it was the direct stimulus of Morgagni's great book.

Théophile Bonet (1620-1689) was born in Geneva, well educated, and in 1643 admitted to the doctorate of medicine in Bologna. Soon afterward he became physician to the Duc de Longueville, and settled down to quiet practice, with abundant leisure for scholarly reading. An accident having rendered his hearing defective, he retired from practice about 1675 and devoted the rest of his life to a gigantic self-assumed editorship of the medical discoveries of the past two centuries, and particularly those made through post-mortem examination, which form the subject matter of his Sepulcher.

He seems to have been a serious soul and patient toiler, with no greater ambition than service to others, for he states in opening the *Sepulchretum,* "This work has cost me as much fatigue and care as the reader will draw advantage from it, but I hope I shall receive thanks for having taken the first step in a career so eminently useful." The work itself is a weighty tome of cumbersome title and 1700 pages, opening with a ponderous dedication, lengthy preface, and imposing list of authors cited, from Hippocrates to his own time. This is followed by several pages of courteous encomium from distinguished contemporary physicians, without which no seventeenth-century work seems to have been properly launched, with Bartholin, Drelincourt, Peyer, Wepfer and others putting in a good word, occasionally in classic meter. Then come a series of cross indices and finally nearly three thousand necropsy protocols with Bonet's own comment and references appended, collected in neat anatomical sections, viz., head, thorax, abdomen, etc., all subdivided into symptomatic sectors, truly a well ordered mortuary.

The great trouble with it is its utter lack of organized deduction. Each case was interesting to Bonet for its own sake in its correlation of morbid symptoms and organic change, but Bonet frankly mistrusted his own capacity to draw general conclusions and left that to others. From it a comprehensive descriptive pathological anatomy, at least, might have been codified, for little that we see today was missed in the stupendous collection. Naturally, a good deal of reconstruction is required for modern interpretation in many cases, and hundreds of the accounts are too brief or obscure for recognition.

The real merit of the work lies in its rediscovery and preservation of the forgotten work of others. Many sections compel our great admiration for the wealth of material collected, if not for its organization. The section on what we now recognize as pulmonary tuberculosis is notable, and much superior to that of Morgagni, who deliberately avoided this disease. Bonet has a hundred pages under the title *De Tabe in genere et Pulmonari,* a vast compilation on the general subject of emaciation. A great many of the cases cited are obviously pulmonary tuberculosis with clear clinical history and convincing, if brief, post-mortem record. In this section Bonet methodically repeats the anatomical changes as revealed by necropsy in case after case in which the outstanding clinical feature was *Tabes,* i.e., severe and progressive emaciation. What is known as consumption today, malignant tumors, and other chronic debilitating diseases are included, more or less indiscriminately. Curiously enough, in the chapter actually devoted to neoplasms (forty pages on *tumores praeter naturam*), he says very little about internal cancer, devoting his attention chiefly to tumors of bones. There is very little on cancer of the stomach, which even Benivieni had recognized, but perforating ulcer of the stomach is recorded.

The treatment of "tumors" of the abdomen, which is chiefly concerned with ascites, is especially interesting. He cited the explanation of ascites given by Richard Lower, who produced dropsy of various regions by ligating the veins from the part (See Chapter XII). Nevertheless he attributed ascites often to disease of the spleen, which for some reason at all times captured the imagination of the ancients. Cirrhosis of the liver came in for surprisingly small attention. There are many records of "nephritis," but they are mostly of the ascending, suppurative type, frequently in the presence of stone. One case from Timaeus is recorded in which the kidneys were "scarcely the size of walnuts."

Not a few gems on diseases of the circulatory organs can be uncovered by search. There is a citation from Richard Lower on what is unmistakably tricuspid endocarditis. There is a clear-cut description of a ruptured aneurysm of the aorta in a university professor 56 years old, who suffered for ten years with abnormal pulsation in the left thorax, taken from the observations of Pietro de Marchetti of Padua (1593-1673). This was presumably a syphilitic aneurysm, not recognized by Bonet as such, in spite of the suggestion on this type of lesion by Fernel and Ambroise Paré. Bonet's own section on syphilitic lesions is very meager, only four pages, devoted chiefly to bone lesions, particularly caries of the cranium, and to "gumma of the dura."

Pneumonia, which Morgagni treated so well, is badly slighted. Bonet is contented to quote Willis, that "peripneumonia is wont to be defined as an inflammation of the lungs, with acute fever, cough and difficult respiration." The acute infections in general are not well described, and it is strange that the plague, which had taken a heavy toll in the two centuries covered, received so little attention.

Summing it up, the work must be recognized as a marvel of

industry, irremediably marred by lack of judgment in grouping and separating lesions, and uncritical acceptance of the cited author's own opinions. It is the greatest collection in the history of pathology, but scientifically no advance on Schenck von Grafenberg.

Two other important compilations of the period are the *Spicilegium Anatomicum* of Theodore Kerkring of Amsterdam (1640-1693), an early associate of Ruysch, and the *Anatomia Practica* of Steven Blankaart of Amsterdam and Leyden (1650-1702). Unlike Bonet, who in all his three thousand cases recorded very few of his own, Kerkring and Blankaart published a relatively small number but from their own experience. About a hundred were collected by the former, including a number of fetal abnormalities and an interesting case of foreign body obstruction of the pylorus. One of the greatest achievements was the recognition of the "polyp of the heart" as a post-mortem product of no significance, a fact that had escaped all pathologists from Benivieni to Bonet. Blankaart recorded two hundred of his necropsies. His descriptions of wounds, pulmonary tuberculosis, carcinoma of the uterus, and dermoid cysts of the ovary are considered by Chiari as well done. There is much that is incorrect and bizarre in addition, however.

These were the texts of pathological anatomy available to the medical profession in 1700. Incomprehensibly, this century of accumulating pathological anatomy passed without a mind to systematize the new knowledge into a science. The material was at hand, but no Galen to organize it appeared. The rarity continued to take precedence over the common in pathological interest. Looking back we see Fernel's *Pathologia* still the most instructive book on the subject, but out of date, and of waning, almost extinct influence.

PLATE X

PLATE IX

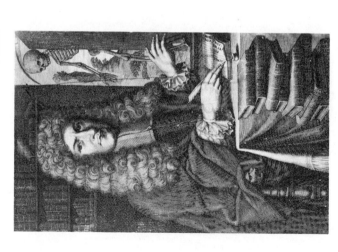

THÉOPHILE BONET (1620-1689)

TITLE PAGE OF *Sepulchretum* OF THÉOPHILE BONET
1679

PLATE XI

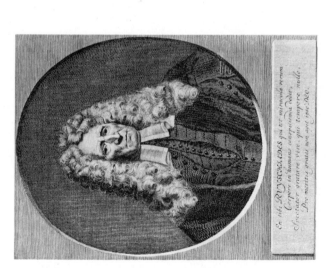

FREDERIK RUYSCH (1638-1731)
Courtesy of National Library of Medicine

PLATE XII

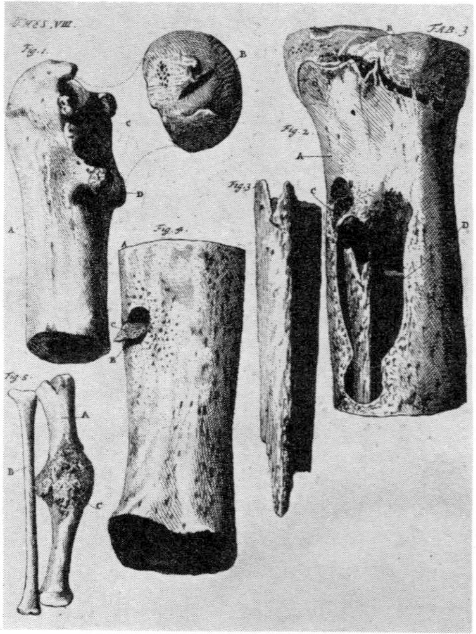

BONE LESIONS
From the *Thesauri Anatomici* of Frederik Ruysch
1724

CHAPTER V

Morgagni and the Eighteenth Century

As we have seen, the seventeenth century opened wide the sources of the growing science of pathological anatomy. Special pathology made substantial advance on the basis of thousands of post-mortem examinations. The most notable contributions were those of Sylvius, Morton and Willis on tuberculosis, and Wepfer on apoplexy, but valuable writings appeared from time to time on tumors, calculi, dropsies, and other conspicuous lesions. Surgical pathology had come into existence in the pioneer labors of Severino and Nicolaes Tulp. In the microscope an instrument of enormous potential value for pathology had been found, and the new media of scientific exchange, such as the Transactions of the recently formed scientific academies, and the published correspondence of men like Thomas Bartholin greatly facilitated the spread of important scientific information.

General pathology, however, had gone astray in the hands of enthusiasts striving for an unattainable system of simplicity. Sylvius (de le Boë) had introduced a new humoral pathology, as incompetent to explain all human ills as the ancient Hippocratic doctrine, while the brilliant young Baglivi and others sought to systematize medical thought in a too simple mechanical conception of the body's action.

The huge compendia of the period, particularly the *Sepulchretum* of Bonet, show the frequency of recourse to post-mortem investigation in general practice, and other records reveal that the necropsy was sought even in the palace. The track of the assassin's knife was mapped with the anatomist's deliberation in the body of Henry of Navarre, and the diarrhoea of the short-lived consumptive, Louis XIII, was traced to tuberculous ulcers, among the first to be recorded, in the royal bowels. At the English court, William Harvey studiously dissected the remains of his noble patients on the principle that "the examination of a single body of one who has died of some disease of long standing is of more service to medicine than the dissection of the bodies of ten men who have been hanged."

Even the layman evinced a keen interest in pathological anatomy. Sandifort tells of a Dordrecht surgeon, one Maximiliano Bouwmanno, who, in recording his necropsy of the daughter of a prominent Brussels citizen, dead of renal calculi and its complications, states that her body *"a me post mortem dissecta est in praesentia plurimarum matronarum."* Evidently the wives of the burghers turned out *en masse* for the event.

Nevertheless, in spite of all its solid achievements, the seventeenth century failed to attain a working codification of this knowledge. Indeed this was finally reached in a form useful to physicians only in the closing years of the eighteenth century in the text and atlas of Matthew Baillie. The intervening years, however, served to extend enormously the range of pathological detail on which such texts might be based.

The departments of anatomy in the continental schools continued to furnish the bulk of this detail. At the opening of the century, the best traditions of the great Dutch school of anatomy were being ably maintained by Frederik Ruysch in Amsterdam (1638-1731), a pupil of Sylvius, with a reputation established even in his student days by his work on the valves of the lymphatics. His chief distinction in later years rested on his ingenious wax injection of all parts of the body, a method of great importance in the understanding of minute structure.

Ruysch advanced pathology by collecting an excellent museum of morbid anatomy and publishing a number of copper-engraved atlases illustrating the collection. His most precious specimens were his skeletons, and the uncertainties of life moved the old Dutchman to grace his works with exquisite engravings of these in quaint postures with lugubrious mottoes, such as *"nascentes morimur,"* an inescapable fact in the daily observation of every pathologist.

Among Ruysch's best specimens were chronic bone inflammations, tumors and other abnormalities, calculi of various types, a large aortic aneurysm (beautifully figured in his *Thesaurus*), stenosing tumors of the rectum, cirrhosis of the liver, carcinoma of the stomach, and a papillary tumor of the urinary bladder (described as "scabies of the bladder with fleshy and glandular excrescences").

In France morbid anatomy was cultivated quite as extensively. Raymond de Vieussens of Montpellier (1641-1716), whose anatomical investigations are commemorated in the "valve of Vieussens" and other structures, in a rich post-mortem experience made notable observations on the pathology of the heart (1715). He clearly described mitral stenosis with calcification of the cusps and dilatation of the right heart, and left an excellent picture of aortic insufficiency in a patient subsequently found to have calcification of the aortic leaflets. In both cases the stagnation of blood flow, or passive hyperemia, dependent on the obstruction, was emphasized, and in the case of the aortic lesion a full pulse was felt, so strong that the "arteries in each arm struck the tips of my fingers like a taut, vibrating string," a discovery anticipating Corrigan by a century.

A celebrated Montpellier graduate, Jean Astruc (1684-1766), professor of anatomy in Paris and later personal physician to kings in France and Poland, wrote important treatises on tumors and venereal disease, as well as a *Tractus Pathologicus* with miscellaneous observations, and a book on diseases of women. Astruc classified tumors meticulously, considering scirrhus a lymphatic development and cancer an outgrowth of "scirrhus," produced through a thickening of the humors. He incinerated a carcinoma of the breast and a piece of ordinary beef-steak, finding the salty residue no more sharp and irritating in the one case than the other, thus disproving in his own mind the ancient theory of malignancy as a manifestation of especial acridity of the humors. He separated true tumors from cysts, which he considered merely dilated lymphatics.

The relation of the lymph system to cancer was being much stressed at this time. Among others, the philosopher and physiologist René Descartes (1596-1650) had emphasized the coagulability of lymph by heat, and the suggestion was rife that cancer could be attributed to its spontaneous coagulation. The great French surgeon Jean-Louis Petit (1674-1750) was calling particular attention to the enlargement of the regional lymph nodes in cancer in support of the lymph theory, and Antoine Louis (1723-1792) even distinguished types of cancer on the basis of the manner of lymph coagulation. Henri François Le Dran (1685-1770), also a Parisian surgeon and particular student of cancer, considered the tendency of cancer to recur in spite of the most careful operative removal, good evidence of an intrinsic abnormality of the lymph.

Astruc's work on venereal disease (1754) is notable for its historical account of syphilis, which he traced to the Americas. His exposition of its contagiousness is excellent and his description of the chancre and second stage of the disease exhaustive. As subsequent lesions he recognized bone and possibly testis involvement, but the characteristic lesions of the aorta and liver escaped him. On the other hand, he ascribed all sorts of ailments, most of them dependent on such general causes as cardiac failure, to the supposed syphilitic virus in the system.

One of the best special treatises of the time is that *On the Structure of the Heart, and Its Action and Diseases* (1749) by Jean-Baptiste de Sénac of Paris (1693-1770), physician to Louis XV. The increase in heart disease with age was noted, and dilatation considered the commonest ailment. Sénac used the term aneurysm of the heart without distinguishing dilatation and hypertrophy. Pericarditis was well described and related to inflammation of the lungs and mediastinum, and hydrothorax was recognized as a manifestation of failing circulation. Sénac was skeptical about the "hairy hearts" and stones and worms in the heart reported in the older writings, and looked upon the polyp of the heart as a formation occurring at the time of death. The germ of the modern idea of septicemia is seen in his conception of pus flowing back into the blood from external ulcers, a view critically considered by Morgagni.

Another light of the Paris school was Joseph Lieutaud (1703-1780), a native of Provence and student of Montpellier, who came to the court of Versailles at the invitation of Senac in 1750, and later attended both Louis XV and Louis XVI. Distinguished already by his studies in normal anatomy, in Paris he cultivated freely a developing taste for morbid anatomy. He included his own most interesting dissections in his *Historia Anatomica Medica* (1767), a tremendous collection of post-mortem observations from the literature of the past, rivalling that of Bonet. The descriptions are objective, but too brief to be useful. The spirit of the reviewer is quite uncritical and etiology is not considered. It is a written museum, collected out of three centuries, and the last of the many books of this class. The edition by Portal is probably the most convenient source today for the necropsies of the sixteenth to eighteenth centuries. For teaching purposes, Lieutaud correlated in parallel columns symptoms and what he considered the usual morbid anatomical basis (as *"Apoplexia—Aqua in cerebro"*), but the brevity of the correlation destroyed its usefulness. It was a monumental work, but out of date the day it came off the press, for the *De Sedibus et Causis Morborum* of Morgagni had already been written.

The Italian school was in its waning glory. One of the most brilliant figures, Giovanni Maria Lancisi of Rome (1654-1720), had passed away, leaving science much enriched by his discoveries in anatomy, pathology, medicine, and hygiene. His two great books, *On Sudden Death* (1707) and *On the Motion of the Heart and on Aneurysms* (issued in 1728), laid the foundation for a true understanding of the pathology of the heart. He distinguished hypertrophy and dilatation (*"aneurysma cordis"*), described thickened valve cusps as hard as cartilage, wrote the first good description of warty vegetation on the valve cusps, correlated dilatation of the heart with syphilis (*"aneurysma gallicum"*) and recognized the relation of heart alterations to valvular stenosis and chronic lung lesions.

Lancisi was also a good epidemiologist. His contemporary and compatriot Bernardino Ramazzini (1633-1714) was equally distinguished in this field. Ramazzini devoted especial attention to the hazards of industry and was one of the first to call attention to the evil effect of the dusty trades on the lungs.

Incomparably the greatest figure of all, however, was Giovanni Battista Morgagni (1682-1771), who culminated the most illustrious line of anatomists of all time in the chair of anatomy at Padua. His teacher was Antonio Maria Valsalva (1666-1723), and it is only justice to the great Bolognese anatomist to state that much of his more illustrious pupil's fame rests on Valsalva's own accurate notations on morbid anatomy. Morgagni himself makes this clear in all his writings, and his edition of Valsalva's works indicates the great regard he had for his master. In the *De Sedibus et Causis Morborum*, it was Morgagni's invariable rule to begin with the necropsies of Valsalva, at many of which, as a matter of fact, he had himself assisted.

Morgagni was born in Forlì, Romagna, and graduated in medicine at Bologna, where he came under Albertini and Valsalva, and later became demonstrator of anatomy when the latter went to Parma. In 1712 the fame of his *Adversaria Anatomica,* his first important book, led to his call to Padua, where he soon succeeded to the chair of anatomy and the most distinguished position on the faculty. Here he remained in a teaching and executive capacity for more than half a century, an extraordinarily popular teacher, a much sought medical consultant, the friend of patricians and Venetian senators, the intimate of Popes, and the recipient of scientific honors from all Europe.

Morgagni's great book on the *Seats and Causes of Disease* was published in the fullness of a long lifetime after sixty years of observation and unhurried thinking. He was seventy-nine years old when it appeared (1761) and he lived to see several reprintings before he died in his ninetieth year.

In his earliest student days, Morgagni made a practice of correlating clinical symptoms with organic change, and this point of view he continued to cultivate all his life. The standard printed work on the subject was the great *Sepulchretum* of Théophile Bonet. The more Morgagni studied this, however, the less satisfied he became, until he finally concluded to supplement it with observations of his own. With this modest intention, Morgagni proceeded to write the work which spelled unintended oblivion for the *Sepulchretum*. The book was written in the form of letters to a friend, who drew him on until Morgagni had written seventy, and in a fashion completed his subject, which was the correlation of the symptoms of common diseases with the underlying pathological anatomy. The letters were then returned to Morgagni, revised, and published in a work of five books.

Morgagni was a Latin scholar of unusual distinction, with a fascinating literary style in no way hampered by a scientific context. With engaging ease he introduces the subjects of his reports as "a certain honest citizen," "a good and pious virgin," "a most powerful monarch," etc. Merchants, lawyers, thieves, highway robbers, priests and nuns, bishops and princes, share his pages. A patrician to the core himself, however, he carried caste distinctions into the necropsy room with him with a steadfastness which only unusual events could upset. For example, we have his case of "a woman of Padua, by name Jacoba, the wife of Angelo Zanardi. Finding thirteen ribs on each side of her body, I enquired out her name and noted it down, something I am not accustomed to do among the common people."

The feature of the work leading to immediate obsolescence of all preceding dissertations on pathological anatomy was its extraordinary completeness of correlation between clinical detail and post-mortem revelation. Pages, not lines, as heretofore, were devoted to the history of the patient's ailment, and the results of the necropsy are recorded at exhaustive length, leisurely, with no apparent fear of taxing the reader's patience. Copious references indicate the author's enormous reading.

Modern pathology properly begins with Morgagni, but it would be a mistake to consider *The Seats and Causes of Disease* a modern text. It is not a book on pathology in the modern sense at all, but is as much a clinical work, with anatomic explanations of disease symptoms. The method of organization is the ancient one by parts of the body and symptoms referable to them. Renal symptoms and gastric symptoms in the same patient split a single case report by a hundred pages. A search for tumor pathology leads the inquirer into every section of the book. Obviously this is not necessarily a defect. Morgagni was, however, fallible like his predecessors. He missed the significance of much that he recorded, and not infrequently stressed matters today known to be incidental, while making but casual reference to associated lesions now recognizable as of the first importance.

His outstanding contribution to special pathology is the exposition of lesions of the vascular system. The dramatic and colorful accounts make of this portion unusually interesting reading. Apoplexy was a subject of prime interest. Morgagni's teacher Valsalva, and Valsalva's teacher Malpighi, and Morgagni's friend Ramazzini, all died of stroke. While admitting the rôle of the small aneurysms of the cerebral vessels described by Wepfer and Brunner, he was inclined to attribute an important part to the choroid plexus in hemorrhage into the ventricles of the brain. He retained the ancient classification of serous and sanguinous apoplexy. His descriptions of the former probably include cerebral infarction, meningitis, and uremia. In one case he describes what was clearly anemic softening ("only the disagreeable odor was lacking to call it rotten"). Paralysis had occurred on the side opposite the lesion, a finding with which Valsalva before him was quite familiar.

The work on aneurysms is magnificent. He was thoroughly familiar with the already large literature on this subject, and left nothing to finish in the way of objective description. He notes that the ancients had no knowledge of aortic aneurysm, "which first began to be known in the sixteenth century." He describes several cases of sudden death from rupture of aneurysms. One case was that of a prostitute whose aorta revealed "in some places the whitish marks of a future ossification, in others small foramina, and in still others parallel furrows drawn longitudinally." An inch and a half above the semilunar valves occurred an aneurysm of "walnut size," which had ruptured into the pericardial cavity. Other accounts detail the cough, air hunger, upright position in sleeping, anginal pains and other

symptoms of a failing heart, in patients with large aneurysms of
the ascending aorta. He stated that in no class of people did
these aneurysms occur as commonly as in guides, postilions and
others continually on horseback, but he refers frequently, like
many predecessors, to a possible relation with syphilis, today
universally accepted.

Rupture of the heart itself is described also, without recognition of the predisposing cause. Vegetative endocarditis is excel-
lently described, one well recorded case occurring as a complication of virulent gonorrhoea. Morgagni devoted considerable
attention to venereal diseases, making no etiological distinction,
however, between gonorrhoea and syphilis. He made the common mistake of attributing to syphilis all the lesions occurring
in the body of a sufferer from this disease, stating that "four
parts, the lungs, aorta, kidneys and their appendages, are found
injured in those who have suffered considerably and for a long
time with the lues venerea." In another summary he asserts that
"we have shown that the lungs are frequently injured in the
lues venerea, and the aorta is sometimes injured from the same
cause, and dilated into an aneurysm." Some of the lung lesions
described are apparently the result of pressure by aneurysms on
the main bronchi, with chronic bronchitis and unresolved
broncho-pneumonia. It would be a mistake, however, to suppose that he established convincingly the syphilitic origin of
saccular aneurysms of the aorta, or considered syphilis the sole
or even usual cause. The great writings on heart and aortic
lesions by Corvisart, Baillie and Hodgson appearing in the next
half century give scant attention to this suggested origin.

Strange as it may seem, the common ailment lobar pneumonia
was a neglected and confused subject up to Morgagni's time.
Morgagni left it an open book. Some of his case histories are
masterly descriptions. For example, a Paduan nun was "seized
in the night with fever, with which she first shivered, and was
cold through her whole body, and after that grew hot. After an
interval of twenty-four hours a pain on one side of the breast
was added to the fever, with a cough quite dry and a hard pulse.
Death occurred on the seventh day." Morgagni confidently
urged, "let the body be dissected; it will certainly be found that
the lungs have the substance of liver." The necropsy revealed
heavy, consolidated lungs, covered with a thick, white membrane, and on section the lungs were found to be of a dense
compact substance like liver, sufficient evidence to Morgagni
that "inflammation of the lungs had been the cause of her

death" (The quotations are based on the translation by Benjamin Alexander, London, 1769). After Morgagni the descriptive term "hepatization" was used routinely for this anatomical picture.

Hardly a phase of pathological anatomy within the range of naked-eye observation was left untouched, and as a rule little interpretation is required for conversion into modern terms. The published record covers about seven hundred necropsies, the majority from Morgagni's own hand and the rest by Valsalva or other friends. In passing, it should be noted that Morgagni grasped the concept of contagion and was extremely careful about exposing himself unnecessarily. He refrained from opening the thorax of a wool-comber, whose symptoms seem to have been those of pulmonary anthrax; he insisted that the bodies of prostitutes lie a certain length of time before dissection; and, like Valsalva, he avoided the corpses of consumptives. The discussion of pulmonary tuberculosis is accordingly one of the weakest sections of the work. Examination of his records indicates that he did open phthisical bodies unwittingly, while at least one case recorded as phthisis is a case of metastatic tumor. Most of the material on phthisis is in the section "On the Spitting of Blood."

Tumor pathology is scattered, but includes some excellent descriptions of cancers of the stomach, rectum, and pancreas. He explains why tumors of the last named organ are difficult to recognize during life, and cites Valsalva's acumen in recognizing cancer of the rectum by the clinical history. A tumor of the adrenal (*"ren succenturiatus"*) is noted, and other references are probably to carcinomas of the prostate and esophagus. He had no idea of metastasis, but described nodules in the liver which are obviously secondary tumors. A number of accounts of cystic tumors of the ovary with ascites are given. He seems to have seen all the common tumors.

Other good descriptions are of cirrhosis of the liver, renal calculi, which must have been extremely common, atrophied kidneys, hydronephrosis with stricture of the ureter, and what is unmistakably typhoid fever ("ulcers to the extent of two hands' breadth next to the caecum, the regional lymph glands grown out into a tumor and the spleen three times the natural size," and he adds, "I have frequently seen the spleen enlarged after other fevers"). Nevertheless, his explanation of many of these lesions was entirely a fanciful, humoral one, often quite bizarre from the modern point of view. Etiology has always been the weakest side of pathology and Morgagni was only like his predecessors and successors in this respect.

His inestimable service to the science of pathology was his emphasis on detail and thoroughness. He was never hurried in a description. He introduced nothing new in the way of method and made few out and out discoveries. In no way did he revolutionize pathology as did Bichat and Virchow. But he improved existing knowledge in every field he touched. After Morgagni pathological anatomy could never again be slipshod or cursory. The new standard was too high.

Morgagni's most distinguished pupil was Antonio Scarpa of Modena and Pavia (1747-1832), whose triangle in the thigh remains a standardized obstacle for freshman medical students. In pathology he is remembered for his investigations on arteriosclerosis, and the distinctions he made between true and false aneurysms (1804). Other contributions of note were on the pathology of bones and perineal hernia. John Hunter, Haller and Sandifort were actively engaged about the same time in unraveling the intricacies of inguinal hernia, while the sciatic type was being described by the Dutch anatomist Pieter Camper (1722-1789).

Another Hollander, Eduard Sandifort of Leyden (1742-1814), ranks almost with Morgagni in the breadth of his observations in pathological anatomy. Pupil and successor of the great anatomical illustrator Bernard Siegfried Albinus of Leyden (1697-1770), he carried his preceptor's methods into morbid anatomy, added pathological specimens extensively to the Leyden museum, and published a beautifully illustrated work under the title *Observationes Anatomicae-Pathologicae*. Among the best records are ulcerative aortic endocarditis, patent interventricular septum, renal calculi, hernias of several types, bony ankyloses and congenital malformations. Cruveilhier called him "the father of iconography in pathology." A compatriot, Andreas Bonn of Amsterdam (1738-1818), a surgeon and anatomist, brought out an illustrated treatise of great value on the pathology of bones.

During all this period while anatomical pathology was making slow but lasting progress on the basis of laborious dissection, system after system of speculative general pathology arose to achieve a bright but transient glory. One of the most prominent of these was the "tonus" theory of Friedrich Hoffman of Halle (1660-1742), in which the ancient doctrine of spastic and relaxed states was supplemented with the newer iatrophysical philos-

PLATE XIII

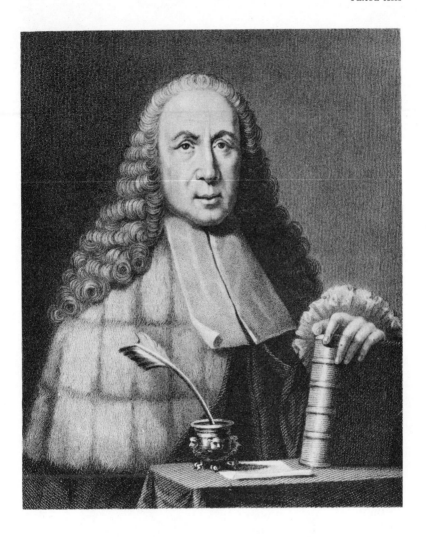

GIOVANNI BATTISTA MORGAGNI (1682-1771)
Courtesy of National Library of Medicine

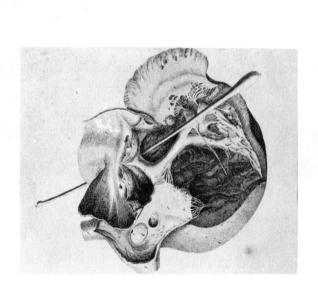

PLATE XV

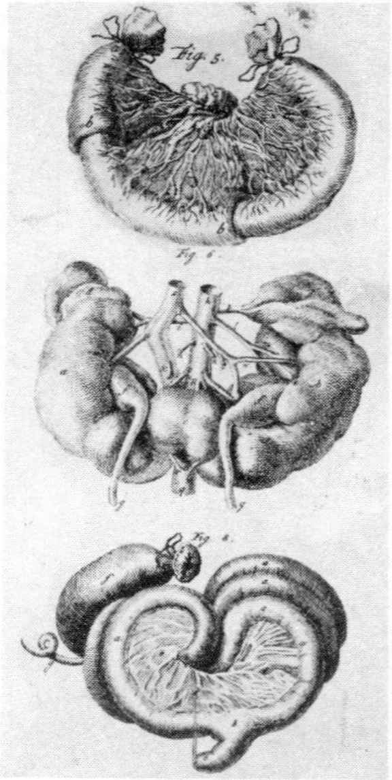

FETAL AND CONGENITAL LESIONS
From the *Observationes Anatomicae-Pathologicae*
of Eduard Sandifort, 1784

PLATE XIV

HEART WITH ENDOCARDITIS AND PERFORATE
INTERVENTRICULAR SEPTUM
From the *Observationes Anatomicae-Pathologicae*
of Eduard Sandifort, 1784

ophy, and the special conception of a nerve force circulated from the meninges, keeping the human machine in proper motion. Without this movement putrefaction occurred, manifested by various symptoms. Fever followed spastic contraction of the nervous and vascular system. Many of these abnormal states were believed to result indirectly from primary dysfunction of the alimentary tract, and a certain amount of permanent good came from the investigation of diseases of the gastro-intestinal system stimulated by this hypothesis.

An equally popular system emanated from a colleague of Hoffmann on the Halle faculty, Georg Stahl (1660-1734), who developed a system something like that of van Helmont, in which the Soul functioned as did van Helmont's head Archaeus. According to Stahl the symptoms of disease were manifestations of the Soul's effort to protect the body against ill. When the natural tendency of the blood to putrefy became threatening, the Soul promptly increased the rate of circulation and excretion, fevers of various sorts arising in the process. If proper circulation failed to occur, a state of plethora developed, leading to gout, concretions, jaundice, etc. Stahl's system of "Animism" conflicted sufficiently with the concepts of Hoffmann to make their close association uncomfortable, so that finally the former moved to Berlin (1716), where he remained as court physician to the end of his life.

The leading authority of the century in general medicine was Hermann Boerhaave of Leyden (1668-1738), called by Haller the "teacher of all Europe." His pupils included Haller himself, Gaub and the great leaders of the "Old Vienna School," van Swieten and de Haën. Boerhaave's own most enduring contribution to science was the conception of "chemical affinity," which has lasted to our own time.

He appreciated thoroughly, however, the value of postmortem examination, and left two remarkable accounts of autopsies from his own experience (*Atrocis nec Descripti Prius Morbi Historia*, 1723, and *Atrocis Rarissimique Morbi Historia Altera*, 1727). In each case the patient was a nobleman whose illness had proved baffling and Boerhaave repeatedly stressed the fact that only through post-mortem examination was it possible to solve the puzzle. His own eminent position apparently secured ready acquiescence from the families in his request for permission to make the inspection. The first case was that of the Baron de Wassenaer (1723), in whose body a rupture of the esophagus was found, with an opening into both pleural cavities. The second case was that of the Marquis de St. Alban, who died from the effects of a previously unrecognized mediastinal tumor.

His pupil and successor in Leyden, Jerome David Gaub (1705-1780), was likewise noted as a chemist, but as the author of the *Institutiones Pathologiae Medicinalis* exerted a powerful influence on European medical thought. This book was in the hands of most medical students, and for a time probably far more widely read than the *De Sedibus et Causis Morborum* of Morgagni. Gaub was as much concerned with "signs of health" as signs of disease, thought of disease as a material entity, and considered each particular disease as having its individual predisposing state, which he referred to as its "morbific seed." On such highly speculative premises the basis for advance was altogether lacking, and Gaub's once widely read text of general pathology was soon forgotten after his death.

At this time the phenomenon of irritability, to which Glisson had directed attention a century before, was becoming recognized as of fundamental importance in physiology, and Albrecht von Haller of Bern (1708-1777), the most distinguished pupil of the Leyden school, went far to develop the modern concepts of muscle irritability and nerve stimulation, on the basis of his exhaustive experimental work at Göttingen, where he spent his best scientific years. This eminent physiologist, whose name is almost as well known to the sciences of botany and anatomy as to physiology, did not omit pathological anatomy from the sphere of his prodigious labors, as did so many of the other great medical systematists of the century. Haller's observations appear in his *Opera Minora*, which include the *De Monstris*, with much good teratology, and the *Opuscula Pathologica*, in which he gives brief objective records of his own more interesting post-mortem examinations, covering a wide range of pathological anatomy, but scarcely adding anything new to the subject.

The phenomenon of irritability, much less exactly considered, furnished the basis for the medical philosophy of the Scottish physician John Brown (1735-1788), a poorly educated but arrogant genius, whose effrontery was coldly met at home, but achieved incredible recognition abroad. Benjamin Rush followed his system in America, and in France Brown's theories were brought to the attention of the National Convention, while in Germany and Austria "Brunonism" had a big following. The Brunonian system of medicine was very simple, as systems unhampered by detailed medical knowledge are apt to be. In brief, "excitability" was the controlling factor of life, moderation spelling health, while excess or deficiency meant disease, to be treated by specific, corresponding regulation of the exciting stimuli. Stimulation so violent as to exhaust excitability or insufficient to provoke it resulted in death of the individual. The system, thus made to embrace all problems of health and disease, seems too fanciful and ill-supported by fact to be taken seriously today, but was of tremendous vogue in its time, and a generation after its origin important enough to be revamped and pushed to new absurdities by Broussais.

These were the men with whom Morgagni competed for the attention of medical Europe, and it must be confessed that in their time the facile systematists were the more popular. It was only with the intense development of pathological anatomy coming with the materialistic French Revolution that Morgagni's stimulus became powerful.

CHAPTER VI

The Paris School at the Opening of the Nineteenth Century

The eighteenth century had seen the peak of anatomy in the great Dutch and Italian schools. The job of gross anatomy was almost done. Gross pathology had kept the pace, but had much farther still to go. Specialists, however, had already come. Two Frenchmen, Vieussens and Sénac, and an Italian, Lancisi, had published invaluable monographs on diseases of the heart. Above all, the century had brought Morgagni, who had covered the whole range of pathological anatomy, and laid his experience before the medical world in one of its greatest classics. General medical thought, nevertheless, continued to be molded in the ephemeral and speculative systems of Hoffmann, Stahl, Gaub, and Brown, touched with a saving dash of the real from the greater systematists Boerhaave and Haller.

In France the Revolution wiped the slate clean for a fresh start. The old medical colleges were abolished, and their faculties disbanded. "Free" societies of medicine replaced the anathematized "Royal" Society. And a new, hard materialism insisting on analytical observation, forcing theory to square with practice, soon brought France to the top rank of the scientific world. No science received a greater impetus than did the investigation of disease. France succeeded fertile Italy, in the words of Cruveilhier, as "the classic land of pathological anatomy."

The hospitals, with the enormous mortality of those septic times, provided an unlimited source for pathological research. The old Hôtel Dieu was a sink of pestilence. In 1788, when Jacobus-René Tenon published his memoirs on Paris hospitals, it was crowded beyond description, most of the patients sleeping four or six to a bed, with hundreds lying on filthy straw pallets in the corridors. Surgical and maternity wards reeked with the stench of pus and gangrenous flesh. Contagious cases were improperly isolated, and veritable epidemics of erysipelas swept the hospitals.

Out of this, in the opening years of the nineteenth century, came, if not an understanding of human ills, at least a clearer correlation than ever before of symptoms and underlying organic change. An industry surpassing belief pervaded all medical instruction. Masters and pupils were in the wards at daybreak. Students finished their day's work late at night, completing in their bedrooms the dissection of noisome specimens from the day's post-mortems. The most brilliant clinical teachers the world had ever seen carried the triple load of care of the sick, clinical instruction, and painstaking dissection of the dead, burning out their strength in a fever of investigation. Two above all others in this manner brought pathology to new ways, Marie-François-Xavier Bichat and René-Théophile-Hyacinthe Laënnec, whose combined span of years reached but seventy-six.

They were respectively the pupils of the two great teachers of the late eighteenth century Paris school, Philippe Pinel (1745-1826) and Jean Nicolas Corvisart (1755-1821). Pinel, whose fame today rests chiefly on his reforms in the treatment of the insane, was a great systematist; his *Nosographie Philosophique* achieved an enormous popularity. Internal diseases were methodically docketed in six main classes, embracing twenty-one orders and eighty-four genera, a short-lived division which would have brought its author no lasting recognition had he not touched the spring which opened the way for Bichat. Pinel classified inflammations into those of (1) skin, (2) mucous membranes, (3) serous membranes, (4) connective tissues, and (5) muscles and joints. It was the first attempt to show similarity in diseases in a given type of tissue, and out of it Bichat created general anatomy and histological pathology.

Corvisart was the greater clinical teacher and left a longer line of immediate disciples, the most distinguished of whom was Laënnec. Corvisart made physical diagnosis the keystone of the practice of medicine. Through his teaching and example, he formed the connecting link between Auenbrugger, whose book on percussion he translated, and Laënnec, who made the physical diagnosis of chest lesions an exact science. Corvisart's own most impressive published work, aside from this translation, was his *Essay on the Diseases and Organic Lesions of the Heart and Great Vessels* (1806). In this he distinguished as "aneurysms" of the heart an "active" form of enlargement with dilatation and hypertrophy, and a "passive" form with dilatation without hypertrophy. He wrote extensively on aneurysms of the aorta and their cause, but did not mention syphilis, which on the other hand he considered important in the production of vegetations on the heart valves.

In 1793 a minor episode of the Revolution brought to Paris Marie-François-Xavier Bichat (1771-1802), whose eight years of work in the capital, in which he brought histology to the service of pathology, established his place with Morgagni and Virchow as one of the trio of founders of modern pathological science. Bichat, born in Thoirette, France, began the study of medicine in Lyons in 1791 under Marc-Antoine Petit and soon became his assistant. In 1793 the Revolution brought him into military service. Difficulties with a badgering officer led to a hurried departure from home, followed not long afterward by the abandonment of military service and a journey to Paris, where he became the favorite student, later the warm friend and colleague, and finally the scientific executor of the great surgeon, Pierre-Joseph Desault (1744-1795). After the latter's death, although he completed and edited his master's surgical works, Bichat turned his attention more to the fundamental branches of medicine, anatomy, physiology, and pathology.

Impressed by the work of Pinel, he began the studies leading to his famous *Treatise on Membranes* (1799-1800), in the light of which he is today looked upon as the founder of histology. A prodigious worker, whose only relaxation was change of labor, unhalted by ill health, carrying a heavy load as teacher of students and hospital physician, he followed his first publications rapidly with his equally famous *Physiological Researches on Life and Death* (1800), and his huge *General Anatomy* (1801-2), one of medicine's greatest books, and his *Descriptive Anatomy*, which was completed posthumously by colleagues. A sufferer from tuberculosis all his working life, he died in 1802, after a particularly trying day, from what appears to have been some form of meningitis. Béclard states that after dissecting a horribly nauseous specimen he fell on the staircase of the Hôtel Dieu and became unconscious. "A violent affection of the head, severe gastric symptoms, and continual tendency to stupor and ataxic symptoms succeeded rapidly, and Bichat died on the fourteenth day of the disease," at the age of thirty-one. Possibly he was the victim of tuberculosis meningitis, the anatomic nature of which was not recognized until Papavoine's distinction of *arachnitis tuberculeuse* in 1830.

Fortunately his message to the scientific world had been delivered. He had carried his ideas on anatomical structure without hesitation into general pathology, and was himself unmistakably aware of the influence they must have upon that science. "The more we examine bodies," he declared, "the more we must be convinced of the necessity of considering local disease not from the standpoint of the compound organs, which are rarely affected as a whole, but from the standpoint of their different textures, which are almost always attacked separately."

His lasting reputation is based on this division of the body into textures, to which he was led partly through an ingenious analogy with chemistry. "All animals," he says, in the *General Anatomy*, "are an assemblage of different organs, which, executing each a specific function, concur for the preservation of the whole. These in turn are made up of many textures of different kinds, which really compose the elements of these organs. Just as chemistry has its simple bodies, uniting to form compounds, so anatomy has its simple tissues which by their combination make up organs." He then proceeded to distinguish twenty-one tissues, including nervous, "cellular" or connective (so-named from its vesicular structure on inflation with air), vascular, muscular, osseous, cartilaginous, absorbent, glandular, dermoid, and others. In all this he did not use a microscope, but dissected by hand with fine tools or, as he states, "submitted tissues to the action of various chemical reagents as heat, air, water, acids, alkalies, salts, desiccation, maceration, putrefaction, boiling, etc., fixing with precision the limits of each organized tissue."

Function lay at the base of all his concepts, which he brought together under a majestic doctrine of vitalism. No groping mystic like Paracelsus and van Helmont, he assigned a specific vital property or different mode of vitalism to each of the tissues he had defined, which he credited with their own type of sensibility and contractility. Disease and death he attributed to a breakdown of these vital principles; life and health to their maintenance: *"La vie est l'ensemble des propriétés vitales qui résistent aux propriétés physiques, ou bien est l'ensemble des fonctions qui résistent à la mort."*

His memorable exhortation in the introduction to his *Descriptive Anatomy* might fitly stand as his own epitaph: "Dissect in anatomy, experiment in physiology, follow the disease and make the necropsy in medicine; this is the three-fold path, without which there can be no anatomist, no physiologist, no physician."

Bichat's last course of lectures was on pathological anatomy. The record reaches us through the manuscript of a devoted follower, the anatomist Béclard, transcribed in turn apparently from the notes of a student in the course. These lectures should be read today for their picture of the existing state of knowledge in pathological anatomy, but, impressive as they are, as written down they do not represent Bichat. In the passage through inferior hands the erudition and spiritual force of the *General Anatomy* have disappeared. The student's note-book could not reproduce the master. As the book stands, familiarity with a wide range of pathological lesion is indicated, but Bichat's special pathology was unquestionably far more extensive and much more accurate than as represented. The work is particularly valuable as a record of Bichat's organization of the subject, even if woefully incomplete in detail. It is, however, not on his special pathology that we must judge Bichat in any event, but upon his doctrine of tissues and their changes, which formed the bridge between Morgagni with all his predecessors and the cellular pathology of today.

One of the major problems of special pathology to which the French school gave especial attention was pulmonary tuberculosis. Two of Corvisart's pupils went a long way forward in its understanding, Gaspard-Laurent Bayle (1774-1816) and Laënnec. Both were consumptives themselves. Bayle, whose *Investigations on Pulmonary Phthisis* appeared in 1810 after years of study at the bedside and on the autopsy table, selected fifty-four cases for special record. He distinguished six kinds of pulmonary consumption, of which chronic ulcerative tuberculosis was by far the most common. The other five pulmonary lesions (and their modern equivalents) were "granular" (miliary tuberculosis), "melanotic" (anthracosis), "ulcerous" (pulmonary abscess and gangrene), "calculous" (encapsulated, calcified tubercles), and "cancerous" (true tumors). He improved on all previous descriptions of the tubercle and its relations to the tuberculous cavity, and he emphasized the relation of chronic ulcerative tuberculosis of the lungs to tuberculosis of other organs, as the larynx, intestine and mesenteric lymph nodes. Although tuberculous phthisis in his day was commonly considered a degenerative sequel of eruptive fevers, acute diseases of the lungs, or syphilis or diseases of the heart, Bayle contended strongly that it was an

PLATE XVI

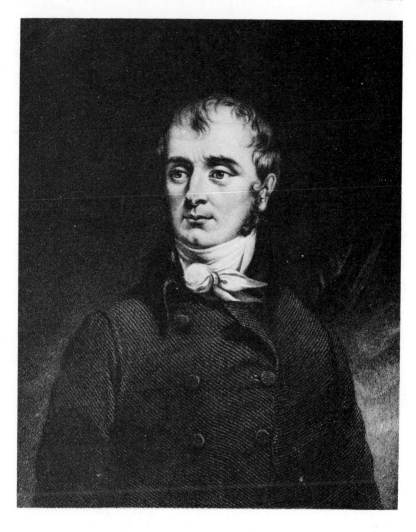

MARIE-FRANÇOIS-XAVIER BICHAT (1771-1802)
Courtesy of National Library of Medicine

PLATE XVII

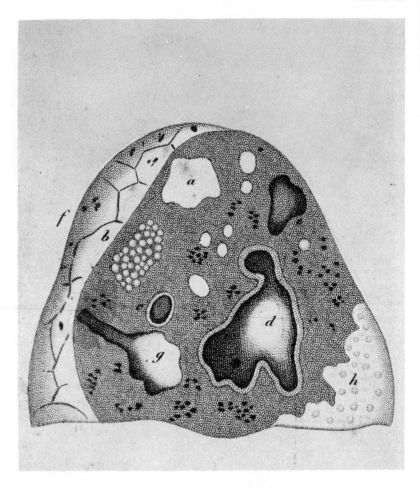

TUBERCULOUS LUNG
From the *Treatise on Diseases of the Chest* of René-Théophile-
Hyacinthe Laënnec, 1823

independent degeneration, the result of an individual tuberculous diathesis.

His more celebrated successor in the field, René-Théophile-Hyacinthe Laënnec (1781-1826), the famous discoverer of the stethoscope, made a masterpiece in the field of tuberculosis incidental to a reform of the whole subject of lung pathology. A native of Brittany, he was a medical student at Nantes when only fourteen years old, and at twenty in Paris already recognized as a man of distinction. The leading teachers in Paris were Corvisart at the Charité and Pinel at the Salpêtrière. Laënnec joined Corvisart and his young assistant Bayle. He also took courses under Bichat, who influenced him profoundly, and under the anatomist and surgeon Dupuytren, with whom he subsequently had bitter differences.

His first publication was on "ossification" of the mitral valve of the heart. He continued to devote his major interest to diseases of the chest, in which he became the recognized authority. His great work on *Mediate Auscultation*, which appeared in 1819, has been called the most influential book on diagnosis ever published. It was reëdited shortly as a *Treatise on Diseases of the Chest*, and in these two books and his articles in the *Dictionary of Medical Sciences* we find most of the material on which his everlasting fame in pathology rests. Like Bichat, he refused to admit ill health as a bar to industry, and his indefatigable labors were terminated by consumption in 1826. No physician has been the subject of more devoted biography than Laënnec.

In addition to his masterly development of the subject of pulmonary tuberculosis, he left unsurpassed descriptions of emphysema of the lungs, lobar pneumonia, bronchiectasis, pulmonary edema, gangrene and infarction (pulmonary "apoplexy") and of hydatid cysts of the lung. Most of the terminology of the succeeding generation in lung pathology and diagnosis, and much that persists today, was Laënnec's. His teaching on cancer of the lungs was the best in his time, and although he referred to the condition as a "degeneration," his real conception was of a substitution of pathological tissue for the normal. In every field he carried Bichat's ideas on tissue individuality into practice. He pointed out that "scirrhous" tumors, on which all predecessors had laid such stress, were not specific tumors of a hard type, or early tumors, but a variety in which much connective tissue made the tumor firm. He followed Bayle in his terms for the soft, brain-like substance of other cancers *(encephaloid, matière cérébriforme)*, which achieved a wide and prolonged usage. Both Bayle and Laënnec considered the concurrence of cancer in two organs, as the stomach and liver, as evidence of a constitutional cancerous diathesis.

Laënnec's most notable contribution to pathology was his unravelling of the mysteries of tuberculosis. He accepted Bayle's contention as proved, that tubercles were not the consequence of preëxisting inflammation, but felt that Bayle had failed to understand their development, none the less. Laënnec followed the tubercle from the tiny, gray, seed-like form, through the larger conglomerate and softening mass to the cavity, proving the essential identity of these dissimilar lesions. He introduced the concept of unity in tuberculosis, identifying the tubercle as the unit. He recognized ages as well as stages in the process. Like Bayle, he considered the disease the result of an inborn constitutional defect.

His work on the heart, also notable, was a much needed supplement of Corvisart. It was written only after exhaustive study of the literature. He was thoroughly familiar with what Bonet, Morgagni, Haller, Peyer, Sénac, and others had written on the subject. It should be noted in passing that Laënnec was a scholar and accomplished medical historian. Because of total failure of correlation with other evidence of syphilis, he disagreed with Corvisart on the venereal nature of the vegetations of endocarditis, which he considered organized "polyps," and he left a splendid description of aneurysms of the aorta, in which he distinguished accurately between the saccular type in the arch and the dilatation in the abdominal portion, without committing himself on the etiology of either form.

Another pupil of Corvisart, and a great admirer of Laënnec, Pierre Bretonneau (1778-1862), did almost as much for diphtheria, to which he gave its present name, as Laënnec had done for tuberculosis. The best previous description was by John Fothergill (1712-1780) of London. Bretonneau recognized the profoundly toxic nature of diphtheria, commenting on "the disproportion between morbid alterations and their fatal results" as a revelation of the weaknesses of pathological anatomy. His contribution to the subject of typhoid fever ("dothien-enteritis") was little less noteworthy. He located the lesions in the patches of Peyer, and suggested a contagious origin.

The subject of typhoid fever was most ably handled in France, however, by Pierre-Charles-Alexandre Louis (1787-1872), another of the great clinicians who for years divided the greater part of each twenty-four hours between the wards and the post-mortem room. Louis had a profound influence through his American pupils on American medicine, and it was one of these, W. W. Gerhard of Philadelphia (1809-1872), who finally separated typhoid fever from the common and more or less similar typhus. The general opinion was that one disease was concerned, with a frequent but not invariable tendency toward ulceration of the small bowel. Gerhard, returning to Philadelphia after two years with Louis, who had published a monumental series of *Researches on the Typhoid Affection or Fever* in 1828, found many cases of the same affection in the Pennsylvania Hospital, to which he became attached, and three years later was actively engaged in the control of the Pennsylvania typhus epidemic of 1836. Examination of 214 cases made it clear to him that he was dealing with something quite distinct from the disease with the intestinal ulcerations, which formed the major part of Louis' report, and his published opinions received almost immediate acceptance abroad.

Louis introduced a new method into the investigation of disease, viz., statistical study of large series of cases. It is hard to believe the fact that this course, now considered of self-evident value, was at first scouted for its novelty. Gerhard, in one of his letters, wrote that Louis was "remarkable for the strict mathematical accuracy by which he arrived at his results," adding that he was "not a brilliant man, not of the same grade of intellect as his colleague at La Piété, Andral." Louis applied the statistical method particularly well in the correlation of symptoms and organic changes found at necropsy in tuberculosis.

We are indebted again to Gerhard for a pithy description of the dean of medical practice in Paris at the time, François-Joseph-Victor Broussais (1772-1838), who comes down to us from Gerhard's pen as "the best known physician of Paris, of universal reputation, who had conferred immense benefit on medicine, but a wretched lecturer." Although himself the author of a general text of pathology, Broussais was too one-sided in his views to be of lasting influence in the subject. He laid gastro-enteritis at the basis of all fevers and most other disorders. He opposed the philosophy of John Brown, then at its height, with regard to sthenic and asthenic states, contending on the basis of clinical observation that one disease could produce both conditions, but in therapy his own influence was absolutely pernicious; his teaching inspired bleeding and leeching on a scale hitherto unapproached.

The fashion in bleeding gave Broussais' successor in the chair of General Pathology and Therapeutics in Paris, Gabriel Andral (1797-1876), the means to pursue an invaluable study on the composition of the blood. An acquaintance with the chemist Jean-Baptiste Dumas and active association with another chemist, Jules Gavarret, supplied the necessary technical assistance. Following Dumas' methods and advice, Andral and his chemical associates analyzed the blood in many different pathological states for the proportions of corpuscles, fibrin, and serum solids. Their figures are not useful today, not of the lasting importance of Bostock's, Richard Bright's associate, on nephritis, which had appeared somewhat earlier, but the work is especially notable for its distinction between primary or "spontaneous" anemia and the secondary anemia from severe or prolonged hemorrhage. Andral recognized, among other causes, lead poisoning as a cause of anemia. The anemic state was measured through the diminished total volume of the corpuscles in the blood and not by counting corpuscles, as today.

Andral was aware of the usual diminution of fibrin in fevers, attributing the enlargement and softness of the spleen in febrile states to this disorder, but emphasized the now well known reverse condition of the blood in pneumonia. He noted that fibrin was low in diseases with a tendency to hemorrhage, like scurvy and typhus fever. The work was well controlled by repeated examination of normal blood, and altogether is entitled to the distinction of being the first extended work of importance on blood chemistry, although the authors carefully cite previous work on the subject. Andral did not confine his attention to hematology, but wrote a number of widely used texts of general pathology.

Although the subject of pathological anatomy was pursued more diligently in Paris than elsewhere on the continent, the first chair specifically assigned to this subject was in Strasbourg in the French province of Alsace, and its incumbent, Johann Martin Lobstein (1777-1835), a native of Giessen, Germany. His success and point of view in anatomy and obstetrics had led Cuvier, the great French comparative anatomist, whose influence extended far beyond the domains of his own science, to recommend the establishment of the position for Lobstein. From the material thus afforded Lobstein started, but never completed, an atlas rich in personal observation. Much more important, he devised a classification of pathological lesions based on the anatomical character of the change, rather than its location, which subsequently impressed Rokitansky.

The final establishment of a chair of pathological anatomy in Paris was due to the insight of the able if ill-natured Guillaume Dupuytren (1777-1835), surgeon-in-chief at the Hôtel Dieu, a pupil of Bichat, and himself a vigorous student of pathology. His careful descriptions of fractures, dislocations and contractures give him a prominent place in the history of its surgical branch. Through his enormous practice he accumulated a large fortune, with a portion of which he endowed the chair of pathology in a legacy.

The new position was conferred in 1836 on Jean Cruveilhier (1791-1874), a pupil of Dupuytren, at the time professor of anatomy in Paris. It is interesting that Cruveilhier, whose eighty-two years witnessed many thousands of post-mortems, was so horrified at the first he saw that for a time he left his early medical studies to return to his original inclination for the church, and actually entered a theological seminary for the necessary training. His father, a physician, soon brought him back into medicine, however, and no further relapse occurred. He graduated in Paris in 1816, his thesis being an *Essay on Pathological Anatomy in General,* an ambitious enough study for a beginner.

His interneship was passed in the Hôtel Dieu in the dark early days of 1814 when Napoleon was gambling the man-power of France against the weight of Europe. Cruveilhier left a vivid description of hospital conditions at the time. The Hôtel Dieu was full of wounded soldiers, and it was here that he developed his famous, if erroneous, notions on inflammation. "For more than six months all wounds without exception, even the lightest, even those on the point of cicatrizing, became involved by gangrene." He added the "remarkable fact" that while gangrene raged in the surgical wards, typhus swept the medical, and was forced to believe in some sort of miasmatic contagion.

After a few years of practice of medicine and a brief tenure as professor of surgery in Montpellier, he returned to Paris to succeed Béclard as professor of descriptive anatomy in 1825. This position he exchanged in 1836 for the new professorship of pathological anatomy, while he acted at the same time as physician-in-chief to several hospitals, including the Maternité,

Salpêtrière and Charité, where he built his teaching in pathology on an enormous post-mortem experience.

Very early in his professional residence in Paris he commenced the work for which he is chiefly remembered, his beautiful lithographed atlas, published, as he says, "to fill a gap in the science, to make pathological anatomy popular, and give the students permanent standards for comparison." The first volume was in the course of publication from 1829-35 and the second from 1835-42. The lithography was largely the work of an experienced illustrator of normal anatomy, Chazal, whose objective spirit and faithful reproduction of important and perhaps at the time little understood detail, made the figures of value lasting even to our own time.

In the days of his youth, Cruveilhier developed a concept of pathology which still dominated the experience of his maturity. It was that tissues were inalterable by themselves, that they were susceptible only to increase or diminution in their nutrition, and that all apparent organic alterations of texture were merely the expression of morbid as opposed to normal secretion within the interstices of the cellular tissue, by an extraordinarily empowered capillary bed. The most important sections of his great *Treatise on General Pathological Anatomy,* which appeared in five volumes between 1849 and 1864, were largely built around this doctrine, and on it he staked the success of his much discussed theory of inflammation, which received its death blow from Virchow.

Inflammation, in his view, was characterized by hyperemia with capillary stasis, and a pathological secretion from the capillaries themselves, which might be coagulable lymph, pus, caseous, or other material. As secondary characters he added an increase in volume and a notable modification in the density or cohesion of parts. He considered inflammation the commonest of all morbid change, and the property of becoming inflamed indissolubly linked with the living state. "That tissue," he contended, "which does not respond by inflammation to stimulants, whether external or internal, in a word all tissue not susceptible to inflammation, is not endowed with life." The immediate seat of inflammation being the capillary bed, which Cruveilhier considered in reality part of the venous system, inflammation of the veins, or phlebitis, came to occupy the most important place in Cruveilhier's views, and in his article on the subject (1837) in the *Dictionary of Medicine and Practical Surgery* he frankly committed himself to the doctrine that *"La phlébite domine en*

PLATE XVIII

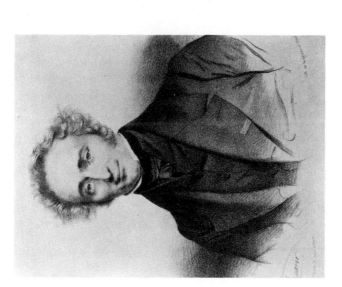

JEAN CRUVEILHIER (1791-1874)

PLATE XIX

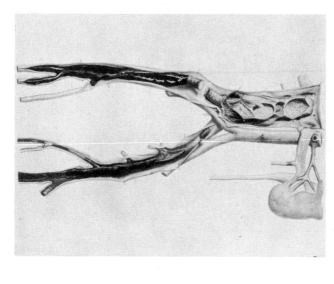

THROMBOPHLEBITIS
From Cruveilhier's *Anatomie Pathologique du Corps Humain*, 1829-42

PLATE XXI

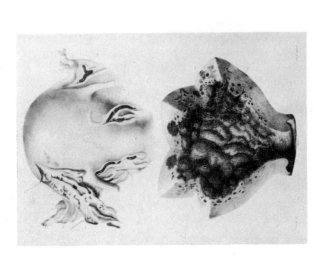

ULCERATION OF THE INTESTINE
(IN TYPHOID FEVER)
From Cruveilhier's *Anatomie Pathologique du Corps Humain*, 1829-42

PLATE XX

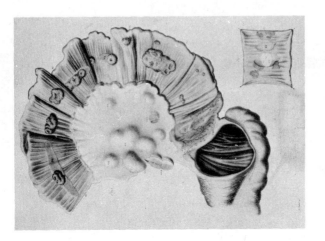

SEPTIC INFLAMMATION OF THE UTERUS
From Cruveilhier's *Anatomie Pathologique du Corps Humain*, 1829-42

quelque sorte la pathologie tout entière." He considered it "the link between the instinctive humoralism of the ancients and the rational humoralism of the moderns."

In spite of his distinction of adhesive phlebitis (or thrombosis) and suppurative phlebitis, that terrible condition with which he grew up in the pavilions of the Hôtel Dieu, he failed to appreciate the possibilities in his concept, and embolism remained unrecognized and pyemia unexplained. Sterile as this doctrine was, on the whole, it permitted Cruveilhier to recognize tuberculosis as an inflammatory condition of a chronic sort, which had hitherto been denied. But he was carried away again in the subject of cancer, to speak of a cancerous juice entering the blood and penetrating the tissue of the various organs. This was the best explanation of the phenomenon of cancer metastasis possible before the cellular pathology and the doctrine of embolism.

A number of excellent treatises in special pathology were brought out by contemporaries. Pierre-François-Olive Rayer (1793-1867) was the author of two atlases of note with accompanying text, and a well-known treatise on human glanders. The first atlas was on skin diseases (1826-1827), and the second accompanied a three volume monograph on diseases of the kidney (1837-1841), appearing ten years after Bright's classic publication. It is the first great work stressing exhaustive analysis of the urine in the diagnosis of kidney lesions. Much attention is paid also to the sediment and microscopic examination for pus. The third volume is devoted to pyelitis, with most of the causes of which Rayer was quite familiar. His strong historical instinct is indicated by copious references to ancient work and views. Rayer is memorable as the writer of the first *History of Pathology*, which formed the subject of his thesis in 1815.

The line of great French writers of monographs on diseases of the heart, which included Vieussens, Sénac, and Corvisart, was ably continued by Jean-Baptiste Bouillaud (1796-1881). He attributed fever to endocarditis, and like Laënnec opposed the Corvisart view that syphilis led to vegetations on the heart valves, finding their occurrence rare in syphilitics and frequent in others. On the other hand, he "would not wish to deny the influence of syphilis on the great vessels," a cautious admission strengthening the vaguely growing suspicion of this disease as a cause of aortitis. His descriptions of stenosis of the valvular orifices are good. His most notable contribution to pathology, however, was his recognition of the relation of rheumatism and heart disease, which was first reported in his *Clinical Treatise on Articular Rheumatism and the Law of Coincidence of Inflammations of the Heart with This Disease* (1840). He also shares with another Frenchman, Paul Broca (1824-1880), the first statements on injuries in the frontal lobe of the brain as a cause of aphasia.

An American-born Frenchman, Philippe Ricord (1800-1889), whose parents were residents of Baltimore, more than any other man helped to solve the puzzle of venereal diseases. Misled by John Hunter (next chapter), conservative European physicians had almost come to accept the etiological identity of gonorrhoeal urethritis and the hard chancre, different as the lesions were. Unsatisfied younger men and particularly the always courageous medical students were, however, still industriously inoculating each other with gonorrhoeal pus and serum from syphilitic chancres by the Hunter method, and an unbelievable amount of human inoculation from chancres was being practiced either for diagnostic purposes, or as a therapeutic measure, both in syphilis and in diseases other than syphilis, on the theory that the two diseases might be "forced to combine" and subsequently be promptly wiped out together by the specific mercurial treatment of syphilis. Ricord in Paris, a man of tremendous diligence and keen powers of observation, through the assemblage of records from such tests, supplemented by an enormous inoculation experience of his own, carried out in a scientific spirit with first solicitude for his patient's interests, was able to separate the diseases beyond question. At the same time he established certain immunological principles on the basis of difficulty in reinoculation, and his descriptions largely served to crystallize our present stereotyped classification of three stages in the disease.

CHAPTER VII

Pathology in England in the First Half of the Nineteenth Century

While French pathology after the Revolution was making the rapid strides described in the last chapter, an equally productive and quite independent movement was under way in England. This period properly begins with the Hunters, who created the first English museums of pathology, and their nephew Matthew Baillie, who brought out the first atlas.

Before them, to be sure, a few physicians like Samuel Clossy (1763) and Richard Browne Cheston (1766) had already published on the subject of morbid anatomical change as correlated with disease, John Fothergill had written the original authoritative description of diphtheria (1748), and a group at St. Bartholomew's Hospital had brought a luster to their institution which was dimmed only by the greater subsequent glory of Guy's. In this group were William Heberden (1710-1801), whose name is inseparably attached to the first clinical description of angina pectoris, published in 1768, and Percivall Pott (1714-1788), the celebrated surgeon whose original investigation of angular curvature of the spine (1779) led to our present designation "Pott's disease" for this condition.

Pott as a matter of fact did not recognize its tuberculous nature, and was less concerned with the lesion itself than the palsy and deformity that might be associated with it. The tuberculous character was established by the French orthopedic surgeon Jacques-Mathieu Delpech (1777-1832) of Montpellier. Pott is remembered also for his work on diseases of the rectum and testis, and for the particular fracture of the fibula bearing his name, which he had sustained himself.

William Hunter (1718-1783) of Lanarkshire near Glasgow, a pupil of Monro *primus* and intimate of William Cullen, was from the outset of his medical career a skilled and informed anatomist. He began practice as a surgeon in London, but soon specialized in obstetrics, in which he made a lasting mark. He was the outstanding London teacher in an age when there were no properly constituted medical schools, and students attended private courses given by men of reputation. Hunter left a long line of brilliant pupils, the most illustrious of whom was his own brother John, who came down from Lanarkshire in 1748 to assist him. Differences over the matter of credit in their joint work led to a highly lamentable quarrel and their lasting separation. Different as day and night in their personality, William polished and restrained, John brusque and bad-tempered, they nevertheless cultivated identical scientific tastes. Both were famous teachers of normal and pathological anatomy, both were life-long collectors of specimens for teaching purposes, and both established museums of morbid anatomy which formed a standard for the medical world. But the younger brother went far ahead of the other in his constant recourse to experiment to back his views, and is commonly ranked the first great experimental pathologist.

John Hunter (1728-1793), the child of his father's old age, brought up by an indulgent mother, was an opponent of convention and conventional teaching from the start. No idler, however, he cultivated freely an absorbing taste for collection of specimens in natural history from his first step to the day of his death. At twenty he moved to London to begin medicine under his brother William, where his ability was immediately apparent. He was soon in charge of William's dissection room, and later his partner. From time to time he took brief service under leading surgeons like Cheselden and Pott, laying the technical foundation for his own later surgical practice, and he made an honest but not prolonged effort to acquire the intellectual culture of Oxford, but the dead classics had no persuasion for his independent, questioning spirit.

After his separation from William he set up establishments of his own in London and the country. With every free moment afforded from his surgical practice and consultation he collected specimens, so that his town house was soon a museum and his country estate a veritable zoo. No living or dead subject of interest to him was safe from his scientific avarice. He was successful in the surreptitious capture of the body of a well-known giant during the actual course of the funeral, and out of his own pocket he financed an Arctic expedition to bring him marine specimens from Greenland. In 1760 he accepted the opportunity afforded in the Seven Years' War to become staff surgeon on the expedition to Belle Isle. During the reduction of the fortress he found time to write his views on the subject of inflammation, which, hitherto unpublished, were, as he felt, being put forth as their own inventions by students to whom he had lectured. The Belle Isle campaign gave him the opportunity to test his ideas on inflammation and furnished the material for his celebrated treatise on gunshot wounds.

Hunter's vast accomplishments resulted more from his unquenchable industry than any innate brilliance. His daily routine was heart-breaking. Up at six, he dissected regularly until nine, then breakfasted and was at home to patients until noon. After that, outside consultation kept him busy until dinner at four. With an hour's rest he was back in his study and laboriously engaged in animal experiment or writing until two in the morning. Out of these long evenings of labor and his daybreak investigation came the two studies of greatest moment for pathology, that on *Blood and Inflammation,* which was published in its matured form together with his study of *Gunshot Wounds* in 1794 (posthumously), and his treatise on *Venereal Disease* (1786).

Like most illustrious pre-Darwinian biologists, Hunter was a zealous teleologist, who saw almost conscious effort in each of Nature's adaptations, a point of view of immeasurable value in his study on inflammation. The concept of "life of the blood" dominated his picture. He was led to this by its notable resistance to putrefaction, as well as its clotting capacity, which so often served the useful purpose of controlling hemorrhage. It did not miss his notice that blood escaping in the pursuance of a presumably useful function, menstruation, did not coagulate. When the objection was raised to his theory that the life-destroying act of freezing blood did not remove its capacity to clot, with characteristic energy he froze a piece of muscle and proved that it still could contract.

His beliefs on inflammation were the natural outcome of this point of view. Inflammation was first and above all else a defensive mechanism, and secondly a restorative process. He classified it in three types, the first of which was *adhesive*. The favorable effect of this type was exemplified in the pleura, where fibrinous adhesions localized an irritating process. This localization was promptly followed by vascularization "giving powers of action to the new tissue." Hunter credited the local tissue with the capacity to initiate this vascularization, quite independently of the general circulation, an idea meeting no serious objection before the development of cellular knowledge.

If the adhesive inflammation failed to control the irritating injury, one or both of the other forms, *suppurative* and *ulcerative*, supervened. He considered suppuration always of inflammatory nature, at the basis of which lay a change in the vascular structure whereby there were separated from the blood, by a process similar to secretion, the materials constituting pus. A modification of these constituents from their original state within the blood was assumed to take place during passage through the vessel walls. This belief in a secretory capacity of capillaries was later developed by Cruveilhier in his doctrine of phlebitis.

The third type of inflammation, viz., ulceration, was a supplement to suppuration, effecting the removal of the dead matter. His ideas on repair, union by first intention, and regeneration were in the main sound. His discovery of collateral circulation on obliteration of the main vessel to the antler of a stag, but one of his hundreds of shrewd experiments, found immediate practical application in surgery in his own hands.

His inextinguishable scientific curiosity led him to devote his own person to inoculation with the virus of venereal disease. Dipping a lancet in the gonorrhoeal discharge of a patient, he introduced the material by puncture into his own skin. Chancre, bubo, tonsillar ulcer (which he did not attempt to treat "until its nature was ascertained" for certain), and copper-colored rash, in a word all the signs of syphilis, following in rapid succession, he was convinced that gonorrhoeal pus had produced syphilitic lesions and the diseases were identical. Ricord's later experiments proved that he must have injected the two viruses simultaneously.

Hunter left a brilliant progeny of pupils, of whom the most distinguished were Edward Jenner, John Abernethy, who succeeded him in his teaching positions, Astley Cooper, his brother-in-law and assistant Everard Home, who injured his reputation with posterity by appropriating some of Hunter's work after the latter's death, and John Thomson (1765-1846) of Edinburgh, considered the ablest expounder of Hunter's pathology. Hunt-

PLATE XXII

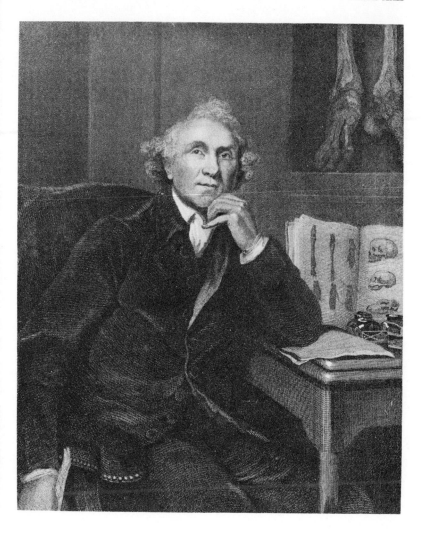

JOHN HUNTER (1728-1793)
Courtesy of National Library of Medicine

PLATE XXIV

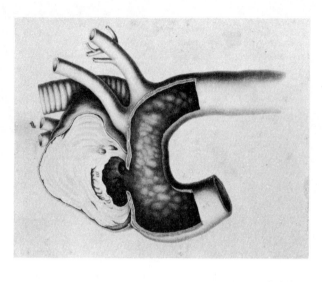

ANEURYSM OF THE AORTA
From the engravings illustrating the *Diseases of
Arteries* of Joseph Hodgson, 1815

PLATE XXIII

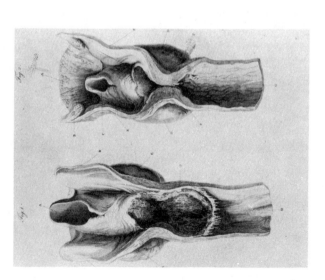

CARCINOMA OF THE ESOPHAGUS
From the engravings illustrating the *Morbid
Anatomy* by Matthew Baillie, 1793; specimens
from the Museums of William and John Hunter

er's most effective teaching was from the cadaver or the living body. He was a wretched speaker, nervously reading his own lectures to his students, and taking laudanum to compose himself. He died of angina pectoris in 1793, twenty years after his first attack, and the necropsy reported by Home disclosed what Jenner had predicted to be the cause of this condition on the basis of his reading of Morgagni, viz., hardening of the coronary arteries. His costly museum, which had profoundly influenced the teaching of morbid anatomy in his time, and had been visited as a model institution by the most distinguished foreign anatomists, went to the Royal College of Surgeons, and shortly after his death an endowment was established for the now famous Hunterian lectures.

The service of the Hunters in the foundation of museums for the teaching of morbid anatomy was extended by their nephew Matthew Baillie (1761-1823), who brought out the first comprehensive atlas of pathology. Baillie also came down from Lanarkshire to assist William Hunter. With his uncles' reputation behind him his course from the start was easy and straight to fame and prosperity. Although a lucrative practice consumed most of his time, his principal interest was in morbid anatomy. His association with the Hunters and access to their museums furnished the necessary material not only for his beautiful copper engravings, but also for *The Morbid Anatomy of Some of the Most Important Parts of the Human Body* (first edition, 1794), to which the atlas formed a supplement. This book is the first text of pathology devoted to that science exclusively by systematic arrangement and design. The demand for such a text was apparent in its immediate extraordinary popularity, necessitating a rapid series of new editions and translations. It was an almost purely descriptive work, with relatively little emphasis on etiology; which does not seem to have been such an acute problem with pathologists as in our time, and perhaps less on associated functional change, although Baillie in his introduction stressed the latter as the real goal in the understanding of morbid anatomy.

There is relatively little citation of the work of others, as compared with the great French monographs soon to follow. Baillie was of course thoroughly familiar with the work on tuberculosis of another Hunter pupil, William Stark (1742-1771), who had made a valuable study of cavities and the cause of hemoptysis, and the sections on phthisis and scrofula are among the most frequently quoted in Baillie's book. The great merit of the work was its simplicity and the clarity with which it brought all the common types of morbid change to the attention of the medical profession.

Baillie's atlas was succeeded a generation later by the *Illustrations of the Elementary Forms of Disease* (1837) by Robert Carswell (1793-1857), who came down from Scotland to assume the position of professor of pathology in the University College of London. This folio of lithographed plates achieved through their color a result unattainable in the copper engravings. Although some are slightly over-tinted, there are good pictures of: postmortem digestion of the stomach, recognized as such; dry gangrene of the toes, attributed in the accompanying text to arterial occlusion by fibrin, fibrous or osseous material; cirrhosis of the liver, with a clearly stated recognition of the accompanying dropsy as due to obstruction of the circulation of the blood through the liver, by contracting tisue; endocarditis, with what Carswell intended to be a refutation of Bouillaud's contention of its inflammatory origin; and tuberculosis of the lungs and intestine, the former showing beautifully that clover-like arrangement of caseous material recently designated "acino-nodular." It is interesting to note that Carswell had never found vessels in vegetations of the heart valves, "although" as he said, "some pathologists state they have succeeded in injecting them." His pictures of carcinoma of the stomach and rectum are fair, but nothing illustrates better than Carswell's annotation of his representation of cancer nodules in the liver, the darkness in this field before the cellular pathology. The liver nodules, obviously metastases, were attributed to a transformation of liver substance through the deposition of a cancerous secretion from the blood, essentially the later Cruveilhier view, as we have seen, and probably the enlightened thought of the time. It remained for the discovery of embolism, and the development of the cellular pathology, to clear the subject. Altogether, however, Carswell's book is monumental, and its relative obscurity and infrequent notice suggest that it was ahead of its time.

Another important English atlas of the same period was that of James Hope (1801-1841), a pupil of Andral. The book (1834) was well received and several foreign editions appeared. Its colored plates, however, are much inferior to those of Carswell and Cruveilhier.

An important monograph appearing somewhat earlier, also extremely well illustrated in an accompanying series of engravings, was the *Treatise on the Diseases of Arteries and Veins*

(1815) by Joseph Hodgson (1788-1869), who was for thirty years surgeon of the General Hospital at Birmingham. It is an erudite work, particularly on aneurysms and their history. Admitting that the disease might commence as a simple dilatation, Hodgson insisted that in its mature form the production of aneurysm always involved the destruction of one or more arterial coats. The work was well received all over Europe, and among the French aortic aneurysm came to be known as *"maladie d'Hodgson."*

We now reach that development leading to England's brightest medical glory, which came about in the hands of a small group of physicians, ever since known as the Great Men of Guy's. In 1725 a London bookseller, Thomas Guy, who had acquired wealth in the South Sea Trading Company, supplemented his previous contributions to St. Thomas' Hospital with a fund for an associated institution, which opened a week after his death as Guy's Hospital. The two institutions continued on cordial terms, St. Thomas' acting as the teaching body, until Sir Astley Cooper (1768-1841), the celebrated surgeon and anatomist, failed in his effort to appoint his own successor in anatomical teaching at St. Thomas'. Mr. Harrison, treasurer at Guy's, came to his rescue with the offer to establish a school there modeled after St. Thomas'. Under the tutelage of Sir Astley Cooper the new medical school flourished immediately.

The development carried with it a tremendous impetus to pathology. Under the old system post-mortems had been relatively infrequent. A physician wishing to make an examination handed in to the steward of the hospital a timid memorandum stating that "a patient in no. — ward being now dead I request permission for the body to be inspected, considering it to be an important case, from which the profession may derive much satisfactory information." Under the later arrangement the post-mortem became more nearly routine, regular staff members were appointed to the service in pathology, records accumulated rapidly, and the museum of morbid anatomy, under a regularly constituted curator, throve as never before. The inspirer of all this, Astley Cooper, who went to bed sorrowfully, by his own statement, if he had failed to dissect something during the day, stimulated the younger men to spend as much time as they could in the post-mortem room.

Under these conditions men of the stamp of Bright, Addison, and Hodgkin grew up. Richard Bright (1789-1858), born to comfortable means, had every facility for study and encouragement in the way of travel and contact with medical leaders. His active career at Guy's, where he had spent part of his student days, commenced in 1820. No man ever stressed more warmly the correlation of the clinic and the necropsy. Although forever memorable for his discoveries in nephritis, or "Bright's disease," he no more confined his attention to the kidney than to any other organ. All pathology drew his interest.

His concern with kidney disease developed through the discovery of its association with dropsy. Anasarca, dropsy, or generalized edema was still thought of as a more or less independent affection, or attributed indifferently to disease of the liver. The association of dropsy and coagulable urine had occasionally been noted, but it remained for Bright to unify the whole story of kidney disease, dropsy, and "albuminuria." This synthesis appeared in his *Reports of Medical Cases* (1827), in which the results of ten years' study are recorded.

Once his attention was called to the intimate relation of kidney disease and dropsy, he had proceeded to separate the dropsies of other origin, and in so doing gave the following clear expression of the relation of circulatory failure to edema: "One great cause of dropsical effusion appears to be obstructed circulation, and whatever generally or locally prevents the return of blood through the venous system, gives rise to effusions of serum more or less extensive." Cirrhosis of the liver, with obstruction of the portal vein and ascites, is given as an example. He also recognized acute peritonitis and tuberculosis of the peritoneum as causes of accumulated fluid in this cavity. In these conditions, however, the urine did not coagulate with heat (the routine test was boiling in a spoon over a candle), and the kidneys were normal.

On the other hand, dropsy was frequently found associated with diseased kidneys, with other organs normal, as shown by his cited cases. Over and over again we meet his description of "small kidneys, rather lobulated, and of semi-cartilaginous hardness," further described as having "small whitish or yellow granules projecting with red intervening spaces, so as to form a scabrous surface, both appearing and feeling rough." And "on making a longitudinal section the kidney cut with the resistance of a scirrhous gland, the tubular part drawn much nearer to the surface than is natural, the cortical part distinctly granular throughout."

In other cases, where the symptoms had been acute, the anasarca was associated with "a large white kidney." Bright felt

PLATE XXVI

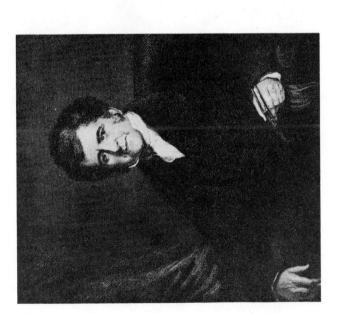

CHRONIC NEPHRITIS
From the *Reports of Medical Cases* of Richard
Bright, 1827

PLATE XXV

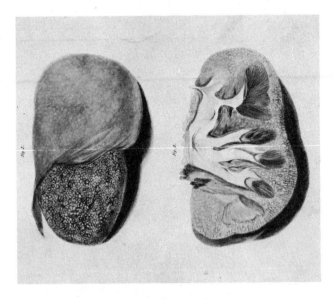

RICHARD BRIGHT (1789-1858)
Courtesy of National Library of Medicine

PLATE XXVII

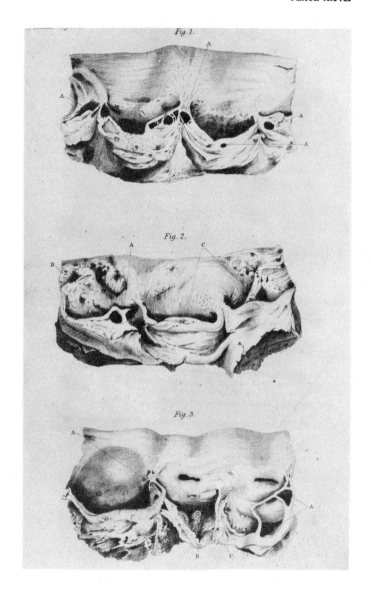

AORTIC INSUFFICIENCY
From the *Permanent Patency of the Mouth of the Aorta* by
Dominic John Corrigan, 1832

reasonably certain he could distinguish three stages of development, beginning with a simple loss of firmness and early mottling, followed by an enlargement with granulation of the cortex and a "copious morbid interstitial deposit of an opake white substance," attended by highly coagulable urine and marked anasarca, and ending with a rough scabrous, hard, contracted organ associated with frequent, but not invariable dropsy. As a matter of fact, in spite of his careful distinction between renal edema and that based on circulatory failure, an analysis of his records in the light of modern knowledge leaves the impression unavoidable that some of his most selected cases were after all examples of cardiac edema with the albuminuria of passive hyperemia, dependent on decompensation of a hypertrophied heart. He noted in his records the frequent coincidence of enlarged heart.

As causes of the kidney damage he stressed intemperance, cold and wetness, with retention of perspiration. He was ably supported in his clinical and post-mortem work by John Bostock (1773-1846) and later by other chemists. Out of this association came the recognition of urea retention in the blood, leading to the concept of uremia, with the present accepted manifestations of which Bright was quite familiar. During this period blood chemistry made great strides, and one of Bright's associates, George Rees (1813-1889), recorded the now well known hyperglycemia of diabetes.

Through the years of his activity Bright contributed frequently to the Guy's Hospital Reports. His last publications were the important series of articles assembled later as *Clinical Memoirs on Abdominal Tumors and Intumescence,* an extremely interesting, learned, fresh, and vigorous work. It opens with a chapter on "exploration of the abdomen" reminding one of the diagnostic teaching of Laënnec. The reports of ovarian tumors and the frequently attendant "ovarian dropsy" are exceptionally able. Another good section is devoted to "acephalocyst hydatids" or echinococcus cysts, which Bright saw frequently in London and in his travels, which had included Iceland, where the disease is endemic today. Many other abdominal swellings are described, although the author made no effort to put out a complete monograph on the subject.

Bright died in 1858, the necropsy disclosing an extensive sclerosis of the aortic valves, with extreme stenosis of the aortic orifice.

A close associate of Bright at Guy's was Thomas Addison

(1793-1860), whose name is inseparably attached to disease of another organ. Like many Englishmen of his time, when London schools were still in embryo, he graduated at Edinburgh. He entered Guy's for further study in 1824, and in 1837 reached the rank of physician to the hospital. Here for many years he was a leading spirit. As his cases multiplied he became more and more interested in a peculiar "idiopathic" type of anemia, not the result of detectable bleeding, with no characteristic morbid anatomy other than a "fatty state of some of the organs." He apparently overlooked the bone marrow. The picture is that of pernicious anemia, often called "Addison's anemia" in recognition of this early description.

In searching for a possible cause, his attention was attracted to a symptom complex, of similar, insidious onset, characterized by anemia, languor, feebleness of heart action, irritability of the stomach and discoloration of the skin, in which disease of the suprarenal capsules was regularly present. His observations on the two conditions were first presented to the South London Medical Society in 1849 and expanded in 1855, with publication of eleven cases. A good descriptive dermatologist as well as pathologist, he delineated the skin changes most carefully. The eleven cases were variable enough in underlying cause to support his conclusion that although the suprarenals were usually scrofulous, malignant tumor or simple atrophy of the glands might lead to the same general condition. He remained confused over its possible relation to his idiopathic anemia. The importance of his discovery was not appreciated until Trousseau in France revived it as "Addison's disease" at a fitting time when internal secretion physiology was developing in the hands of Claude Bernard.

Although never receiving the notice they merited, on account of their obscure publication, Addison's investigations in pneumonia showed keen insight. He correctly attributed the pulmonary consolidation to exudate within the lung acini, not, as prevalently believed, in the interstitial tissue, the existence of which he refused to recognize. All unaware, however, of the dawning cellular pathology, he spoke vaguely of "albuminization" of the lung and "reconversion to a state resembling the albuminous material forming the basis of all tissues." Independently of Rokitansky he clearly distinguished lobular from lobar pneumonia, even recognizing the hypostatic variety of the former, ("mixture of congestion and inflammation") and surpassed Laënnec in his description and understanding of pulmonary atelectasis.

In the midst of all this brilliance the professional pathologist of the hospital, Thomas Hodgkin (1798-1866), was far from being outclassed. As curator of the museum and demonstrator of morbid anatomy he developed the collection enormously, and added to its usefulness by an accurate catalog. He was the first in England to pursue the lead of Bichat, by discussing morbid changes in their tissue aspects, and wrote a monumental treatise on the *Morbid Anatomy of the Serous and Mucous Membranes* (1836-40). Later pathologists at Guy's looked back to Hodgkin as a pioneer.

His name is preserved for the more casual student in that constitutional affection characterized by enlargement of certain groups of lymph nodes and the spleen, commonly called "Hodgkin's disease." As a matter of fact, his two papers *On Some Morbid Appearances of the Absorbent 'Glands and the Spleen* (January 10 and 24, 1832) record cases recognizable as tuberculosis, leukemia, and perhaps secondary neoplasms, as well as the condition now bearing his name. The seven cases reported were from the experience of Bright, Addison, and Carswell, as well as his own, and, as he himself stated, did not record a new disease, but were published simply to call attention to a set of changes hitherto insufficiently noticed.

Failure to secure a promotion in the hospital led to his retirement in 1837 for medical practice, and almost immediate loss to pathology. A member of the Society of Friends, a philanthropist by nature, he later took part in an expedition to the East to render aid to the Jews; there he died of dysentery in Joppa in 1866.

One of Hodgkin's best papers, appearing in 1827, dealt with retroversion and incompetence of the aortic valves. As we have already seen, Vieussens had described this condition, and Hodgson left a magnificent plate figuring it in 1815. Apparently the time had not been ripe, however, for its understanding, and aortic insufficiency is usually associated with the name of Corrigan. Dominic John Corrigan (1802-1880) was a member of the great Dublin school that included the brilliant clinicians, Graves, Stokes, Cheyne, and Adams. His paper on *Permanent Patency of the Mouth of the Aorta or Inadequacy of the Aortic Valves* appeared in 1832. He distinguished the condition from aneurysm, although noting their frequent interrelation, and recognized four types: (1) absorption of patches of the valve cusps,

(2) rupture of the cusps, (3) tightening of the cusps with failure
to spread across the aortic orifice, and (4) dilatation of the
entire orifice. The characteristic water-hammer pulse, which he
correctly attributed to the valvular incompetence, has since
been known as "Corrigan's pulse." He recognized at once that
the hypertrophy of the heart associated with aortic regurgitation
was not a disease but a compensation.

The Irish College of Physicians at first failed to appreciate
Corrigan's merits and voted down his proposal for membership,
but he lived to be their President five successive times before
his death at seventy-eight.

Two important English studies on hematology should be
mentioned at this point, although both were overshadowed by
more exhaustive work in Germany. One was by William Addison (no relation of Thomas), a practicing physician and an early
devotee of the microscope, who in 1843 wrote an article on
*Researches on Inflammation and the Origin and Nature of
Tubercles in the Lungs*, which anticipated Cohnheim by twenty-
five years with regard to many features of the vascular and
leucocytic response of inflammation. Clearly recognizing and
distinguishing the mono- and polynuclear leucocytes, he considered "pus corpuscles as altered colorless blood corpuscles,"
and not, as commonly believed, a development from granules
and molecules of blood in the inflamed tissue.

The other important work was the discovery of that condition
in which the blood is loaded with white cells, by John Hughes
Bennett (1812-1875), pathologist of the Edinburgh Royal In-
firmary, which was recorded in 1845 in an article on *Hypertrophy
of the Spleen and Liver*. He called the disease "leucocythaemia,"
distinguishing it from suppuration, and in later articles, after
Virchow also had recorded the disease, under the name "leu-
caemia," he did much work in its further elucidation.

The greatest English champion of independent teaching of
pathological anatomy, whose broad comprehension of the field
unified its rapid and unrelated developments, was Samuel Wilks
(1824-1911), pathologist of Guy's Hospital, whose long span of
life embraced all the great modern developments in the science.
No other man so well appreciated the work of the great Guy's
group, and no other so lamented the inadequacy of the students'
routine course in pathology. His own lectures in this short
course were so popular that at his students' request he brought
them out in book form in 1859, unfortunately using the Guy's
museum outline rather than a logical organization in presenting

them. He based these lectures on the two or three thousand post-mortem examinations he had himself seen. At this time about two hundred and fifty were being performed annually in the hospital under Wilks' direction. Of Wilks' original contributions perhaps the outstanding was *On the Syphilitic Affections of Internal Organs* (1863), which described gummas of the liver and other organs, and had a good deal to do with the final acceptance of the common aneurysm of the aorta as a syphilitic lesion.

There was no better text of pathology in the English language during this period, however, than that prepared in 1839 by the Pennsylvanian, Samuel D. Gross (1805-1884), professor of surgery at Louisville and later at the Jefferson Medical College of Philadelphia, who gave the first regular course in pathology in the United States. Its three editions met a notable reception not only at home but abroad, where it was commended even by the critical Virchow. It was almost an isolated production, however. With the earlier *Treatise on Pathological Anatomy* of William Edmonds Horner (1793-1853), likewise of Philadelphia, an able contributor to the study of cholera, it formed this country's only home-grown textual material in pathological anatomy. American pathology failed to establish itself in this period, and Americans in quest of training in morbid anatomy continued for years to visit the great deadhouses of Europe.

CHAPTER VIII

Rokitansky and the New
Vienna School

The period described in the last two chapters brought about a notable development of both general and special pathology, which France and England shared on equal terms. The leading French contribution was unquestionably the introduction of tissue pathology by Xavier Bichat. The impetus given to special pathology by the brilliance of Laënnec, particularly in connection with diseases of the chest, and the teaching atlas and text of Cruveilhier were also of profound influence. In England John Hunter had established experimental pathology, Matthew Baillie had brought out a series of engravings and the first modern text of pathology, and an outstanding group of men at Guy's Hospital, headed by Bright, Addison, and Hodgkin, had cultivated several fields of special pathology with great profit.

The tide of rising knowledge was now about to swing eastward. As the high mark was passed in France and England, Central Europe was commencing a development soon to capture the leadership in pathological anatomy, to hold it into present times.

To understand the events leading up to this we must go back a century and pick up a dropped thread. In 1745 Gerhard van Swieten (1700-1772), one of Boerhaave's most able pupils, was invited to Vienna to become personal physician to the Queen Maria Theresa. Here his influence, combined with that of Anton de Haën (1704-1776) of the Hague, who had come to Vienna at the same time, made of the Austrian capital the most notable offshoot of the great Dutch school of medicine. Among the reforms instituted by van Swieten were the establishment of hospitals, development of clinics, and improvement of the

Imperial Library. De Haën seems to have been responsible for and to have conducted the first routine necropsies before the students in the clinic.

One of the most capable members of this Vienna school, commonly called the Old Vienna School in contradistinction to the far more brilliant school of Rokitansky's time, was Leopold Auenbrugger (1722-1809), physician-in-chief to the Hospital of the Holy Trinity, the famed discoverer of the art of percussion in physical diagnosis, which was communicated to the world in the same year as Morgagni's *Seats and Causes of Disease* (1761). Auenbrugger compared his observations on living patients suffering from tuberculosis, pneumonia, pleural effusions, etc., with the revelations at post-mortem, and even made experiments on the dead body, injecting fluid into the pleural cavity and percussing out the fluid level. Most of his precious observations appear to have been made on the bodies of consumptives, but his notions on the nature of this disease were entirely archaic; emotional influences and acridity of the thoracic lymph still played a great part in his views on its pathogenesis. His work was slighted by his associates, and would have been altogether forgotten had not Corvisart in Paris thrown the tremendous weight of his reputation into its revival.

The modern period in Vienna properly begins with the founding of the Allgemeines Krankenhaus in 1784 and the assumption of its directorship by the great sanitarian Johann Peter Frank (1745-1821) in 1795. Attention was called at the time of his appointment to the unusual opportunity in pathological anatomy, and limitations on the opening of bodies were largely removed. About 14,000 patients were passing through the hospital annually at this time. In 1796 the sum of 2559 florins was appropriated for the construction of a morgue, post-mortem room, and living quarters for a prosector.

The new position went to Alois Rudolf Vetter (1765-1806), a native of Carlsbad, educated at Innsbruck and Vienna, whose genius in the face of bitter difficulties was recognized by Johann Peter Frank. Vetter had incurred the animosity of van Swieten's successor Anton Stoerck, and the latter's determined opposition in his anatomical and surgical studies. In spite of this, the gifted youth brought out a *Manual of Anatomy* (1788) and followed it with a text on physiology (1794). In connection with the latter, he was again in difficulties over the proper assignment of credit for certain scientific discoveries.

Relieved temporarily from some of his troubles by Frank's

appointment, although at first without salary, he had his long desired opportunity for unhampered study of disease in the human body. At the age of thirty-eight he could look back on the dissection of several thousand bodies. The museum of pathological anatomy, consisting of four or five pieces at the beginning of his tenure, increased to over four hundred in his hands. In 1803 he brought his observations together under the title *Aphorisms from Pathological Anatomy,* a work with little theorizing, but an abundance of good objective description, particularly in connection with lesions of the gastrointestinal tract and pulmonary tuberculosis.

With coöperation Vetter might have ushered in the great Vienna development, for which the time was ripe, but something in his nature stirred up constant envy and animosity. His *Aphorisms* were poorly received, and before he had the opportunity to make any contributions of lasting importance, he threw up his Vienna position, which kept him in poverty and brought him nothing but unhappiness, to accept a place in Cracow. He returned after a short stay and died soon after.

After Vetter the position sank into insignificance. Peter Frank left the hospital in 1804, and a series of lesser men succeeded Vetter. In 1821 new superintendence brought about a temporary revival. An *ausserordentlich* professorship in the University of Vienna was created for the prosector of the hospital, who was required to handle medico-legal pathology as well as give certain stipulated lectures. The first incumbent in the new régime, Lorenz Biermayer, who had acted as prosector on the old basis since 1811, was at the beginning extremely industrious, but soon had occasion to lament the same lack of coöperation from the clinical men as Vetter. Disappointment and disgust led him first to indifference in his work, and finally to drink, neglect of his duties, and suspension. A reinstatement brought little improvement and in 1829 he was succeeded by his assistant Johannes Wagner (1800-1832), whose brief tenure of office gave every promise of a brilliant career. Wagner's observations on cholera, internal hernias, and other intestinal lesions, however, were interrupted by his early death, and the luckless prosectorship of the Allgemeines Krankenhaus was again open. At this low ebb Carl Rokitansky, Wagner's assistant, came into the position.

Carl Rokitansky (1804-1878), was born in Königgrätz, Bohemia, and studied medicine in Prague and Vienna, where he graduated in 1828, becoming assistant to Wagner in pathological anatomy in the same year. As a student Rokitansky had been

PLATE XXVIII

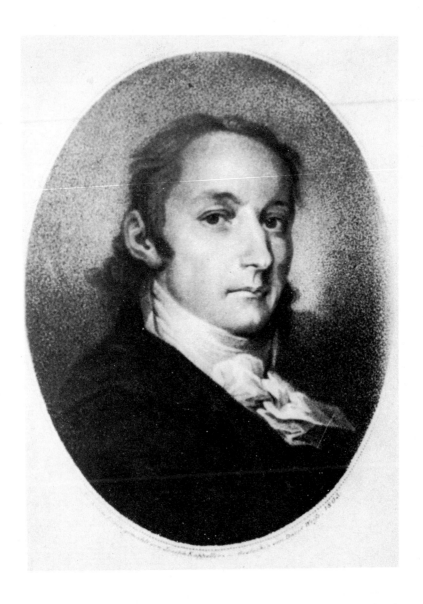

ALOIS RUDOLF VETTER (1765-1806)
Courtesy of Prof. E. Loewenstein

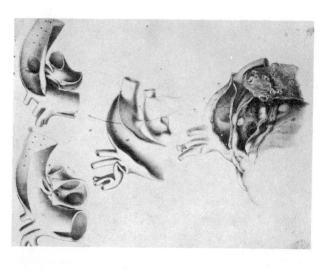

PLATE XXIX

CARL ROKITANSKY (1804-1878)
Courtesy of Prof. E. Loewenstein

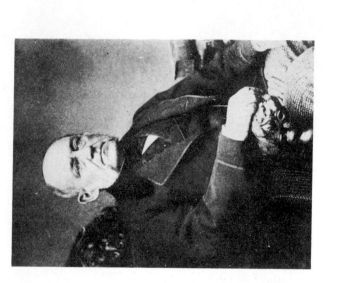

PLATE XXX

CONGENITAL ANOMALIES OF BLOOD VESSELS
From *Some of the Most Important Diseases of
the Arteries* by Rokitansky, 1851

profoundly influenced by the writings of Martin Lobstein and Gabriel Andral, as well as others of the great contemporary French school, and particularly by those of Johann Friedrich Meckel (1781-1833), one of the creators of comparative anatomy. Meckel's embryology had brought about an understanding of congenital malformation, until then the darkest field in pathology, and broken the current tradition attributing "monsters" and all deformities present at birth to malign supernatural influence. This early interest brought Rokitansky into contact with Wagner, and after two years of acting headship of the department, following Wagner's death, he succeeded to the place in his own right. The position remained only that of *ausserordentlich* professor, however, for ten more years, until Rokitansky's growing fame made imperative the creation of a full professorship in pathological anatomy. Under his direction necropsies were performed on an unprecedented scale, averaging 1500 to 1800 a year. Rokitansky wrote his own first protocol on October 23, 1827 and his thirty thousandth in March, 1866.

While this development was taking place, an equally notable revolution on the clinical side occurred. This was largely under the stimulus of another Bohemian, Josef Skoda (1805-1881), a native of Pilsen, of humble antecedents, who worked his way through the university into medicine, and soon attained preëminence in the Allgemeines Krankenhaus. Much impressed by the work of Corvisart and Laënnec, he ultimately replaced a good deal of the empiricism of the French school by an independent classification based still more closely on the actual state of organs as found post-mortem. His own principal contributions were on percussion and auscultation, and his name remains familiar to students today in the term "Skoda's resonance."

Associated with Skoda and Rokitansky in the great development were such celebrated specialists as Hebra and Politzer, the anatomist Josef Hyrtl (1810-1894), and, after 1849, the physiologist Wilhelm von Brücke (1819-1892), a pupil of Johannes Müller. With this multiple origin, and both French and German intellectual stimulus, but independent personal initiative, arose on the decrepit frame of the Old Vienna School a far stauncher new construction, which in a few years was drawing eager students from the entire world. Never before had the fundamental branches of medicine been so actively cultivated, nor with so little regard for the presumable object of medical science, therapy and the relief of the patient. Under Skoda's dominance diagnosis was supreme and the only remaining object of interest

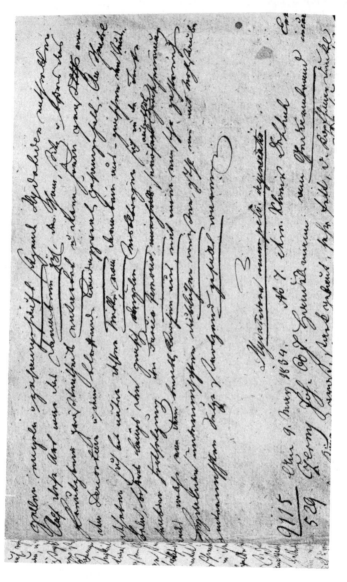

PROTOCOLS WRITTEN BY ROKITANSKY
Courtesy of Prof. E. Loewenstein

was its confirmation at necropsy, which was performed with surpassing thoroughness.

Rokitansky was a first class anatomist, not the least of his service to pathology being the development of a necropsy method which in its anatomical logic and comprehension of detail insured an inspection of every part of the body in every examination. A majority of the many post-mortem methods practiced in central Europe today are simply more or less modified, as their authors freely admit, *"nach Rokitansky."* His procedure combined thoroughness of exposure and inspection with preservation of continuity in structure, differing in that respect from the later likewise thorough and popular method of Virchow, which permitted more separation of anatomic systems. He was far from content, however, with a simple anatomical exposition. His picture of the case included etiology and development of the state finally submitted to view, as well as the functional derangement involved, and even extended to therapy, a field given scant attention by some of his most distinguished associates in the medical clinic. More than any man up to this time he served to establish disease types, with all their varying cause and symptomatology, on an anatomical basis. After Rokitansky names of diseases, like pneumonia and typhoid fever, conveyed to the well trained medical graduate an anatomical picture and not as theretofore, a list of symptoms of varying complexity. This was Rokitansky's undying contribution to medicine.

In view of the magnitude of his task, it is not surprising that, as Weichselbaum put it, "in seeking further explanation he reached into error." Viennese in spirit, if not Vienna-born, he was too much a product of the brilliant Austrian capital to restrain imagination and a dramatic instinct altogether, in shaping his concepts. The ablest descriptive pathologist of his day or any day, he was nevertheless unable to be content with facts demonstrable to his eyes, and built an air castle of theory, which must have been very close to his heart. It was a terrible blow when the less imaginative, harder-headed Virchow demolished it with a single vicious blow.

This untenable doctrine was his famous hypothesis of crases and dyscrases, built out of the newly current physiological teaching of a "blastema," or primitive fluid substance, from which formed elements were derived. With Schwann's new theories (see next chapter) on the cellular nature of life at his disposal, he selected the wrong half for further development and made an altogether misguided, if courageous, attempt to restore humoral

pathology, which had been steadily losing ground since Vesalius
first took issue with Galen. Rokitansky's views are expressed in
the first volume of his great *Manual of Pathological Anatomy*,
which was actually the last volume of the series to be printed
(1846), in which he frankly stated: "Humoral pathology is simply a requirement of common practical sense; it has always held
a place in medical science . . . and of late years has met with a
new basis and support in morbid anatomy."

It is impossible to present Rokitansky's theories in simple
form, so far do they depart from present-day conceptions. His
views remind us of John Hunter's conception of "vitality" of
the blood and, throughout, we see the imprint of Andral's more
substantial quantitative study of blood fibrin in different diseases. All diseased states were referred by Rokitansky in the
last analysis to anomalies of the blood. Moreover, diseases once
localized were capable of engendering further abnormality in
the circulating blood. He felt that chemistry would ultimately
solve most of the difficulties of pathology and "urged upon the
chemical pathologist unremitting prosecution of his researches,"
particularly from a qualitative standpoint, which Rokitansky
believed might explain some of the variations in exudation,
suppuration, and organization of new tissue which he was unable to fathom through unaided anatomical study.

For the time being only, as he indicated, he resorted to an
empiricism, which he hoped would attain ultimate chemical
support, by developing concepts of specific crases, all going back
to an original impairment of the blood, "a primitive affection
of the entire blood mass," with a specific affinity for particular
localizations, e.g., a "croupous fibrin crasis" for the respiratory
system, evinced in diphtheria and pneumonia, a "typhoid
crasis" for the mucous membrane of the ileum, the familiar
typhoid fever, and an "exanthematous crasis," as illustrated in
the common eruptive skin diseases.

He insisted that the dyscrases underlying these organ affections did not always become so localized; a certain degree of
intensity was necessary for this to occur. On the other hand, an
established local dyscrasis did not invariably give rise to a
consecutive dyscrasis of the general circulation; the latter took
place only when a sufficient quantity of the diseased, degraded,
septic, or otherwise modified plasma was absorbed. But in the
main the local and general dyscrasial manifestations were intimately linked.

Once set in motion the theory permitted inexhaustible refinements of classification. Alpha, beta, and gamma varieties of the croupous type of the fibrin crasis were distinguished. Special tubercle and cancer crases were recognized, as well as a typhoid and even a drunkard's crasis, further divided into acute and chronic forms. He spoke with settled conviction of the "expenditure of every atom of tuberculo-dyscrasial fibrin in the formation of tubercle," and wholly in the dark on the subject of pyemia, with which Hunter and Cruveilhier also had wrestled impotently, spoke of "a spontaneous primitive pyemia of the entire blood mass" as well as a "local pus production" dependent on the same crasis. It only required his elaborate conception of interconversions of crases to render the entire doctrine an unintelligible fantasy.

It was this amazing and altogether unnecessary extravagance, upon which the author "confessed to have exercised a certain favoritism" in preparing his great book, that moved the younger Virchow in one of his first published articles to open fire with the full force of his deadly, convincing logic. A "monstrous anachronism," Virchow called it, and so it was, if not worse. After this Rokitansky rewrote his *Manual*, which passed through two more editions, and tried to forget his unfortunate crusade for the lost humoralism in the light of the new cellular pathology.

It must not be supposed, however, that Rokitansky's whole system of pathology fell with his crasial theories. Virchow himself conceded Rokitansky to be the greatest descriptive pathologist of the day, and no mistaken theorizing could detract from the solid merit of Rokitansky's gifted exposition of pathological morphology in the different diseases. Following the system of Lobstein and Adolph Wilhelm Otto (1786-1845), the Breslau anatomist, he comprehended the various lesions to which each organ or tissue might be subject under (1) deficiency or excess of formation, (2) deviations in size, (3) deviations in form or position, (4) interruptions in continuity of structure, and finally, (5) anomalies of texture or content, a system totally ignoring etiology, but permitting convenient grouping in a time when etiology was not well developed. The enormous material of the Allgemeines Krankenhaus ensured the inclusion of practically all known forms of disease under one name or another.

His separation of hyperemia into active, passive, and mechanical forms, directed the later teaching in this subject; his explanation of active hyperemia was entirely in line with the modern teaching on innervation of the capillaries. He consid-

ered active capillary dilatation the primary feature of inflammation, and the subsequent stasis with exudation a secondary,
directly dependent phenomenon of the first importance.

Rokitansky's journal publications, which appeared for the
most part in the *Yearbook* of the Austrian States, the *Zeitschrift*
of the Medical Society of Vienna and publications of the Acad-
emy of Science of Vienna, do not record, by any means, all of his
most significant original discoveries, many of which were given
to the world without any attached claims in his great manual.

His greatest monograph was *The Defects in the Septum of
the Heart,* which appeared separately in 1875, near the close of
his long and busy life, a labor which had occupied his attention
for many years. It served to complete a study of 1851 *On Some
of the Most Important Diseases of the Arteries.* Congenital malformations occupy a good deal of space in each, and in his
obvious special interest in this field we see the lasting stimulus
of the great teratologist Johann Friedrich Meckel. Rokitansky
was a good embryologist and able to predict in advance such
failures of development as might be expected through embryological mischance in one part or another, just as a chemist can
predict the discovery of elements to fill gaps in his periodic
system. Out of his colossal experience Rokitansky was able to
fill all these gaps in the predictable congenital anomalies of the
vascular system. Acquired lesions were, however, not neglected;
his atlas of diseases of arteries figures even such rarities as
the now more frequently recognized periarteritis nodosa.

His special pathology of other organs was scarcely less noteworthy. He extended Laënnec's description of emphysema, improved existing knowledge of pneumonia, distinguishing the
lobular variety and the various stages up through resolution in
the lobar type, described acute yellow atrophy of the liver,
perforating gastric ulcer as a special type, goiter, cysts in the
various viscera, lardaceous disease of the spleen, liver, and kidneys (Virchow's "amyloid"), and acute and chronic inflammation of the heart valves, and wrote at length on neoplasms of
the various organs. True to his humoral hypotheses in his original *Manual,* he attributed tumor growth to the local meta-
morphosis of both solid and fluid blastemata from the blood
stream, fibrous stroma developing out of the solidified blastemata, and cellular and nuclear, as well as fibrous textures from
the fluid blastemata. He used the terms sarcoma and carcinoma,
both familiarized by long usage, not as we use them today nor

quite as they were used in his own time, but as the equivalents of "benign" and "malignant" tumors respectively.

Some seventy thousand necropsy protocols were available to him at the time of his retirement. He lived to enjoy the greatly improved working conditions of his own Institute in Vienna. For the last quarter of a century, he was the outstanding medical figure of the city. His influence was not confined to pathology but was extended to the fundamentals of medical education in general and its curriculum. In 1849 he was made dean of the medical faculty and in 1850 rector of the University. In 1874 a great celebration was held in his honor in which the whole city participated. His retiring statment made clear that he had cultivated pathological anatomy as the most fruitful line of investigation for medicine, and one fundamental to pathological physiology and the elementary doctrine of medicine, and that he considered the logical supplements to pathological anatomy to be pathological histology, chemical pathology, and experimental pathology on living animals, and considered pathology itself not only of service to the practice of medicine but illuminating to biology itself in its broadest aspects. His death occurred on July 23, 1878.

His successor was Richard Heschl (1824-1881), who held the position from 1875-81. Heschl's chief contributions were on amyloid and its special staining characteristics, on pulmonary infarction, and calcification of the ganglion cells of the brain. He was succeeded by Hanns Kundrat (1845-1893), who also had been an assistant to Rokitansky. Kundrat made important contributions on congenital malformations, and described the lymphosarcoma.

On Kundrat's death Rokitansky's heritage began to separate. The direct successor in the professorship was Anton Weichselbaum (1845-1920), who supplemented the more strictly morphological Vienna pathology with the new and rising point of view on etiology. Weichselbaum was one of the first in Vienna to appreciate the part bacteriology was to play, and a pioneer in studying inflammations of the serous membranes in the new light. He was particularly interested in tuberculosis, and a number of his leading pupils, particularly Anton Ghon, have advanced our knowledge in this field.

Other important positions in the pathology of Vienna went to distinguished students of the Rokitansky school. Alexander Kolisko (1857-1918) took over the control of medico-legal pathology for a time, ultimately succeeding Weichselbaum in the chair of pathological anatomy on the latter's retirement. He is noted for his study of sudden death from natural causes, for his editorship of the *Beiträge zur gerichtliche Medizin,* inaugurated on the occasion of the one hundredth anniversary of the establishment of a separate department for forensic medicine in Vienna, and also for an elaborate, accurate study of abnormalities of the pelvis.

Richard Paltauf (1858-1924) succeeded to the direction of the Institute for Pathological Histology and Bacteriology, and later followed Stricker and Knoll as director of the Institute for General and Experimental Pathology. He developed a great talent in the new field of immunology, greatly fostering this science in Vienna. He was influential in establishing the important *Zeitschrift für Immunitätsforschung.* In pathological anatomy he followed the lead of his teacher Kundrat in the study of lymphatic tumors.

During this period the combination of brilliant teachers, with exceptional facilities for study and cordial municipal coöperation, made Vienna the most popular seat for instruction in pathological anatomy in the world.

Intimately related to the Vienna school was that at Prague. Hans Chiari (1851-1916), who had assisted both Rokitansky and Heschl, took the Vienna tradition to this city, where he succeeded Klebs in 1882. His expert technic, the fame of his necropsy method, and his teaching ability brought him many students. The peculiar situation in Prague, where high grade Czech and German universities existed side by side, had always been a source of nationalistic complication. Wenzel Treitz (1819-1872), discoverer of the fossa and muscle bearing his name, as well as the type of hernia associated with the fossa, had taken his own life in melancholic depression over the disputes. Chiari's work likewise at times suffered from the political unrest. In 1906 he succeeded Recklinghausen in Strassburg.

In fields related to pathology the most remarkable achievement of the New Vienna School was the discovery by the Hungarian, Ignaz Philipp Semmelweis (1818-1865), a pupil of Skoda and Rokitansky, of the contagious nature of puerperal sepsis (1847-1849), which confirmed the previous suggestions (1843) of the American, Oliver Wendell Holmes (1809-1894). Semmelweis, as an assistant in one of the obstetric wards in the Allgemeines Krankenhaus, was impressed by the preponderance of child-bed fever in his ward, which was visited by students fresh from the dissection room, and the relative freedom from this condition in the ward devoted to the instruction of midwives. The similarity of the lesions found at post-mortem in the women dying of the fever to those found in cases of blood poisoning from putrid wounds, soon convinced him that the essential causes were identical. His reform of obstetrical practice based on this discovery ranks with the vaccination of Jenner in the annals of preventive medicine.

The leading surgeon of Vienna, Theodor Billroth (1829-1894), a product of the great contemporaneous Berlin school, also took an early active interest in wound sepsis, in which condition he was one of the first to discover bacteria. His great surgical experience with lesions of the alimentary tract went far to complete our knowledge of the pathology of this part, while his intensive studies of the gross and minute structure of tumors, to which reference is made in the next chapter, establish his place not only as a leader in the development of surgical pathology, but also as one of the founders of cellular pathology. He constantly emphasized research in pathological histology as the rational basis for advance in surgery.

CHAPTER IX

Virchow and the Cellular Pathology

As we look back to the middle of the last century, we see pathology in an advanced but curiously helpless state. The major facts in the gross representation of disease had been assembled. Building on the far from insignificant gross pathology of the seventeenth and eighteenth centuries, Lancisi, Valsalva, Morgagni, Sandifort, Senac, Corvisart, Laënnec, Louis, Gerhard, Bright, Addison, Hodgkin, and scores of colleagues and contemporaries had established pictures of disease in the various organs not easily surpassed. The accumulation of isolated details was fast rendering some sort of cementing doctrine imperative. All the systems that had been developed to supply the linking substance, however, soon proved of faulty strength. The vague and imaginative systems of "animism" and "Brunonism," as well as the more tangible doctrines of blood vitality and phlebitis, or inflammation of the veins, emanating from John Hunter and Cruveilhier, proved false or incapable of extension. Only Bichat's monumental work on tissues had helped to clarify the situation, and even that fell short of pathology's needs.

The latest attempt to embrace the specific facts of pathology in a single system, as we have just seen, was that of Rokitansky, under whose touch the faltering Old Vienna School of medicine had quickened into new life. But Rokitansky, a master in the art of description, with a colossal post-mortem material at his disposal, failed worse than all the rest in the matter of generalization. Mature when the cellular doctrine of life was first promulgated, he might have been the first cellular pathologist. The original cellular theory, however, recognized a primitive "blastema" as the source for development of cells, and with tragic misjudgment the great Viennese pathologist selected this un-sound basis on which to build his structure.

It was in Germany, where the cellular teaching was born, that surer hands found in the new knowledge a mold, not for the mere merger but for the reformation of all pathology. The inspiration for this development came from a remarkable man, the last of the philosophers whose learning comprehended all branches of science, the greatest teacher of the nineteenth century, Johannes Müller (1801-1858) of Bonn and Berlin. As the preceptor of Schwann, Henle, and Virchow, he was the source from which both modern histology and the cellular pathology arose. One of the first to use the microscope in analyzing tissue, as early as 1830 he had gone deeply into the histological study of glands and cartilage. Of greatest significance for pathology, however, was his precocious work *On the Finer Structure and Form of Morbid Tumors,* which appeared in 1838, the year in which his pupil Schwann first pointed to cellular growth as the basic principle of animal life. This article established for all time the cellular character of new growths. It was based in turn on his own preliminary studies published in 1836, in which he had distinguished two types of tumor on a semi-histological basis, the *"carcinoma reticulare"* and the *"carcinoma fasciculatum."*

The later work, supported by the recently improved microscope and the chemical methods so useful to Bichat, boiling, treatment with acids, etc., brought to light not only the cells but some of their own minute characteristics, and something of their mode of development. Keenly aware of the inherent possibility of distinguishing tumors on this cellular basis, which has since been realized, Müller compared clinically benign with highly malignant tumors, but found the same structures, viz., cells, internal nuclei, granules, and external fibers in both. His pupil Schwann was at the same time demonstrating those very elements in normal tissues.

So the resourceful Müller sought to bring chemistry to his aid, and succeeded in isolating several types of protein substance, including a colloid which seemed to him to have some specificity, to which he gave the name "collonema." Virchow later identified it with the extract of simple, edematous connective tissue. Müller's treatise was published in an uncompleted form and never afterwards finished. He left it with the cellular character of tumors established and their origin from normal cells presumptive. The distinction between benign and malignant tumors remained of necessity the clinical one of behavior.

Müller's pupil Theodor Schwann (1810-1882), who had studied under the master at Bonn and assisted him in Berlin, after preliminary researches on putrefaction and spontaneous generation, was led into his greatest work partly through an accident. A chance conversation with the botanist Matthias Jakob Schleiden (1804-1881), who established the cellular nature of plants in 1838, stimulated Schwann to take up the cellular study of human tissues, which he had indeed commenced, more intensively. The discovery that all animal tissues were cellular led Schwann to issue the famous generalization: "There is a principle of development common to the most different elementary parts of the organism, viz., cellular formation." His first announcement appeared in 1838, and the fully developed treatise in 1839.

In taking over Schleiden's concepts, however, Schwann carried along a serious error, which Virchow uncovered, but which proved a trap for Rokitansky. This was the "blastema" theory. Schleiden and Schwann believed that in the development of tissue a formative fluid, the "blastema" or "cytoblastema," gave rise first to a nucleolus and next to surrounding granules which condensed to form the nucleus, about which in turn new matter gradually gathered with final condensation into the cell's cytoplasm. In other words, cells were capable of a kind of intracorporeal spontaneous generation. This theory of free cellformation was current teaching until wiped out by Virchow.

Before Virchow's appearance, however, histology was to undergo an almost equally notable development in the hands of another of Johannes Müller's pupils, Jacob Henle (1809-1885), who held the chair of anatomy successively in Zurich, Heidelberg, and Göttingen. It is largely to Henle's early investigations that we owe our present histological classification of tissues. As Garrison says, "the histological discoveries of Henle take rank with the anatomical discoveries of Vesalius." The results of his first investigations were fortunately available to Virchow when the latter was developing his cellular pathology.

It was not alone as an histologist that Henle's genius was expressed. His *Hand Book of Rational Pathology* (1846-53) was a standard text for students. We meet Henle again in connection with the theory of microbic contagion, where his logic did much to bridle an extravagance in the early days of the germ theory fast getting out of hand.

This development of histology found almost immediate appli-

PLATE XXXI

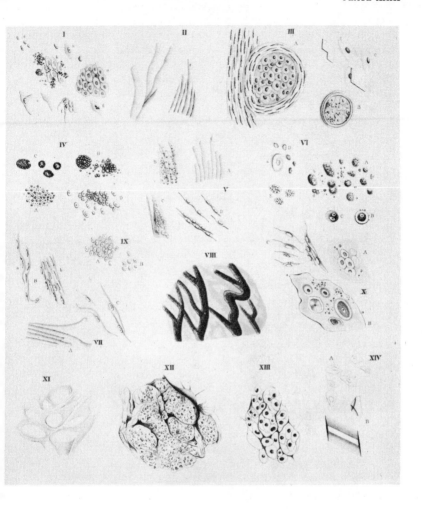

HISTOLOGICAL PICTURES (CARCINOMA)
From the *Icones Histologiae Pathologicae* of Julius Vogel,
1843

PLATE XXXII

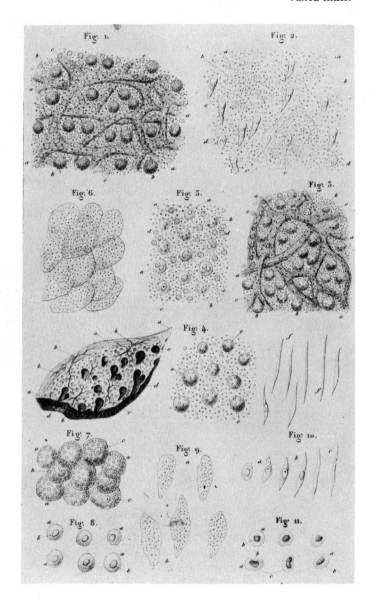

HISTOLOGICAL PICTURES (LUNG DISEASE)
From the *Physiologie Pathologique* of Hermann Lebert, 1845

cation in pathology. Within six years after the announcement of the cell theory two atlas texts of pathological histology had appeared. The first, by Julius Vogel (1814-1880), appearing in 1843 while its author was professor in Göttingen, emphasized the fact that recent developments had made an atlas of pathological histology as necessary as one of gross pathological anatomy. It was divided into two parts corresponding roughly to general and special pathology. The sections for microscopic study and preparation of the plates were cut with a double-bladed knife (see the brief account of the history of histological technic in Chapter X).

The other text came from the hands of Hermann Lebert (1813-1878), a native of Breslau, who led an itinerant existence in Germany, Switzerland, and Paris, publishing his discoveries with equal facility in German and French. His atlas of twenty-two excellent plates, with its attached text, was a product of the Paris period, appearing under the title *Physiologie Pathologique ou Recherches Cliniques, Experimentales et Microscopiques* (1845).

With the circulation of these books and some of less importance which followed, the cellular idea of pathology gradually crept in, and it became customery to speak of the tubercle cell, the cancer cell, etc. But no generalizations of importance were made until Virchow's entrance on the scene.

Rudolf Virchow (1821-1902), the greatest figure in the history of pathology, was a native of the country village of Schivelbein in Pomerania. He matriculated in Berlin in 1839, where Johannes Müller and Johannes Lukas Schönlein (1793-1864) developed in the youthful student a deep interest in the basic concepts of natural science. He graduated in 1843, with a thesis on a phase of inflammation, a broad subject which continued to occupy much of his attention for years to come. Pathological anatomy was at this time relatively undeveloped in Berlin. The leader was Robert Froriep (1804-1861), prosector and curator of the museum at the Charité Hospital, professor of surgical anatomy in the University, and editor of a periodical known as *Froriep's Notizen,* the journal to which Virchow's first articles were contributed. Froriep was an able anatomical illustrator and a voluminous translator of the works of Astley Cooper, Dupuytren, and other leading surgeons.

In the year following his graduation Virchow entered Froriep's service as assistant prosector, where in addition to dissecting dead bodies he cultivated industriously two studies that in his far-seeing judgment were to rejuvenate pathology, microscopic study of tissues and analytical chemistry. In 1846, when Froriep left for Weimar, Virchow became prosector of the hospital. At this time he was in active association with another rising young pathologist, Benno Reinhardt (1820-1852), and with Ludwig Traube, who was later to become the outstanding figure in experimental pathology in Germany. In the year of Virchow's assumption of the duties of prosector Traube started the *Beiträge zur experimentellen Pathologie*, which carried some of Virchow's first publications, with many more in prospect. Its early discontinuation, with only two volumes completed, and the rapid accumulation of important data in the hands of the industrious Virchow and Reinhardt led these youthful investigators to the bold project of launching their own journal, which opened in 1847 as the *Archiv für pathologische Anatomie und Physiologie und für klinische Medizin*. This was a move of outstanding importance. The journal met a hearty reception from the medical profession as filling an obvious need, and has remained the leading journal of pathological anatomy to the present time. With Reinhardt's untimely death it passed into the exclusive editorial control of Virchow, and has since been known by the simple abbreviation "Virchow's *Archiv*."

The following year, 1848, a momentous one for Germany, the Prussian Government sent Virchow to Silesia to investigate a serious epidemic of typhus fever. His report was a masterly compilation of terrible medical and social facts regarding the unfortunate inhabitants of the region studied, but too democratic in spirit for the reigning powers. While writing his report the indefatigable Virchow was also coöperating in the publication of a semi-political journal, *Die medizinische Reform,* and airing views in sympathy with the revolutionary movement then in progress. This was too much, and the young pathologist was removed from his position.

His release in Berlin was the prompt signal for an invitation to Würzburg to assume the chair of pathological anatomy, the first full professorship in this branch in Germany. After seven fruitful years, out of which came the cellular pathology, years which made Würzburg the most sought university in Germany for teaching in pathology, while Berlin languished, the influence of Johannes Müller brought about the establishment of a full professorship in pathological anatomy in Berlin with an invitation to Virchow to return and fill it. In his absence from the city his old friend Benno Reinhardt and, after the latter's

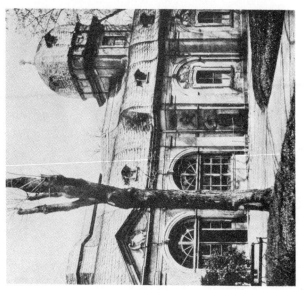

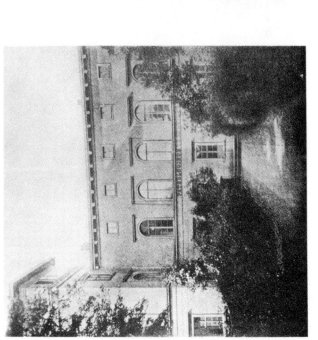

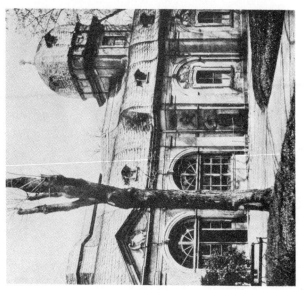

PLATE XXXIII

THE OLD PATHOLOGICAL INSTITUTE IN THE CHARITÉ
Courtesy of Prof. Otto Lubarsch

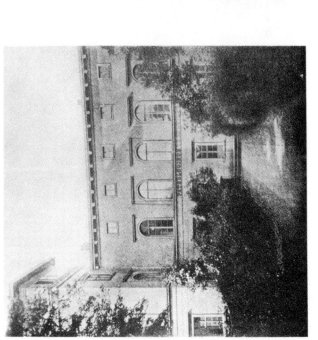

PLATE XXXIV

THE WÜRZBURG PATHOLOGICAL INSTITUTE IN
VIRCHOW's TIME
Courtesy of Prof. Otto Lubarsch

PLATE XXXV

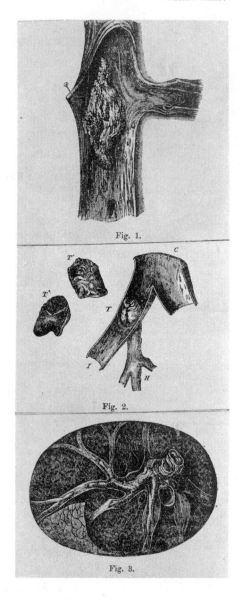

Fig. 1.

Fig. 2.

Fig. 3.

THROMBI AND EMBOLI
From Virchow's *Thrombose und Embolie,* 1846

death, Heinrich Meckel of Hemsbach (1821-1856) for three and four years respectively had held the prosectorship. Back in Berlin, Virchow gave his first attention to the museum of the new Pathological Institute of which he was the director, and bent heartily to those labors which made him the leading pathologist of the world.

The *Cellular Pathology*, issued as a compilation of his own lectures, was one of the first publications of this new period. Much of its content was based on previous investigation, however, which we may now consider. In his earliest days as Froriep's assistant he had squarely taken issue with Cruveilhier's reigning doctrine of phlebitis, or inflammation of veins, as a cause of most pathological lesions. Out of his studies in this field came his classic work on thrombosis and embolism (1846), his solution of the riddle of pyemia, his weighty views on inflammation, and as a side discovery, his recognition of leukemia.

Clotting of blood within the vessels during life was an old story, and its common occurrence in inflammation had led John Hunter and Cruveilhier to relate the two processes intimately. Cruveilhier had carried the matter to the point of believing that all inflammation began with some kind of blood coagulation, and in the frequent absence of demonstrable coagula in the veins, fell back on an hypothesis of "capillary phlebitis." Yet conflicting facts constantly arose, upon the most obvious of which Virchow seized as the starting point of his investigations, viz., the commonly observed coagulation in the absence of detectable inflammation.

He began by comprehending the various phenomena of intravascular coagulation of the blood under the term "thrombosis." Experiment, added to deduction from observation on the dead body, finally led him to conclude that inflammation of the veins was neither the cause nor result of coagulation within their lumen. The coagulation resulted from an entirely different set of causes, of which slowing of the current was by far the most important, whether brought about by compression, abnormal dilatation, general debility of the patient, or other reasons. The thrombi around the uterus, which had so impressed Cruveilhier in the septic maternity wards of Paris, were classed by Virchow in the dilatation group. Before the end of his long, active life he was forced to modify and supplement this original belief considerably, but it had the great merit of clearing the ground for a new start.

The association of thrombosis in one part with the occurrence of abscesses in the lungs was too frequent not to be brought into the study. Central softening of the clots afforded him the clue. Pointing out to his students that shortly after the formation of a clot a central mass appeared, exhibiting a greater or less resemblance to pus, he showed that this softening could and frequently did lead to the detachment of fragments which might be carried along in the blood stream and driven into remote vessels, causing immediate fatality in the case of large masses impacted in the main arteries of the lungs, or lesser consequences from smaller particles. To the detached fragments, whatever their size, he gave the name of "emboli."

Unable to furnish objective proof of small emboli in the "pyemic" abscesses of the lung, he resorted to the statistical method, which Louis in France had found so useful, and confirmed his belief in the "metastatic" nature of these lesions by the study of a large number of cases from a recent severe epidemic of puerperal fever. The regular association of abscesses in the lungs with softening thrombi in the veins around the uterus, and regular absence in just as severe cases where the inflammation was limited to the uterine lymphatics, furnished overwhelming proof that pyemia, a mystery to physicians from the day of its recognition, was a simple consequence of transfer of solid particles from one inflamed region to another point by the direct path of the blood stream, or in Virchow's term, "embolism."

Until the dawn of bacteriology he remained in the dark as to the septic nature of the secondary lesions or metastases, simply noting that if the process at the primary site ran a favorable course, the embolus like the thrombus became converted into scar tissue and pigment, while if gangrenous softening occurred at the original site of the coagulum, the metastatic deposit "assumed the same gangrenous character, just as if gangrenous matter had been inoculated." He also clearly described and explained on the same basis the scattered abscesses associated with the presence of vegetations on the heart valves.

In the study of "puriform thrombi," pus, "pus corpuscles" and their relation to blood leucocytes, he stumbled very early in his studies (1845) on that unrelated condition of overwhelming concentration of white cells in the blood to which he gave the name of *"weisses Blut"* or leukemia. As we have seen, the disease was independently described in the same year by Hughes Bennett. The superficial similarity of this anomaly to inflammation is indicated by the astonished ejaculation of a Berlin physician as Virchow opened the heart in one case, "Why, here's an abscess!" Virchow soon distinguished two types of leukemic affection, which he immediately brought into line with his studies on the formation of the blood, the physiologist in Virchow always keeping up with the pathologist. In one kind he noted that the *spleen* reached enormous size, with moderate but not excessive enlargement of the lymph nodes of the body, while in the other the *lymph nodes* were tremendous, in one case filling the pelvis to such an extent that the rectum and bladder were scarcely visible, while the spleen was only moderately enlarged. He noted, too, that the white corpuscles in the blood differed in the two instances, in the first type being large and "similar to cells of the spleen," while in the other they were small, consisting almost solely of nuclei, and altogether like the ordinary cells of lymph glands. Thus early was our present distinction of splenic (or now splenomyelogenous) and lymphatic forms of leukemia established, one which has required very little modification since Virchow's first descriptions.

The subject of inflammation constantly recurred throughout these studies, and was never absent from Virchow's thoughts. It had been the great sunken reef of pathology on which all systems had foundered. A quarter of a century before, Andral, utterly discouraged, had advised dropping the whole idea of inflammation as an entity. Virchow recognized *irritation* as the invariable cause of inflammation, stating his inability to imagine inflammation without an irritating stimulus, of the nature of which, in those pre-bacteriologic days, he was of course usually ignorant. He cast aside rather brusquely the famous four cardinal symptoms, erecting "lesion of function" as the outstanding characteristic, based in turn upon a nutritional disturbance of the part. He went on to develop the conception of an "inflamed cell," the abnormal state of which he attributed to excessive absorption of fluid and attendant matter under the influence of vascular or other changes induced by the primary irritation. His view thus fixed on that abnormality which today goes under the names "cloudy swelling" and "intra-cellular edema" as the essence of inflammation, an abnormal state of the tissues which might vary with enormous complexity in other respects. He returned to his pre-graduation studies, which formed the subject of his thesis, on inflammation of the cornea of the eye, a structure without blood vessels, to prove his contention that the vascular changes to which predominant attention had always been drawn heretofore, were in fact accessory. His views on inflammation led directly into his cellular pathology, which we may now take up.

As a youth of twenty-five he had wrecked the elaborately conceived humoral system of Rokitansky. His criticism in the *Berliner medizinische Zeitung* of Dec. 9 and 16, 1846, had received the prompt, weighty support of Johannes Müller, and in a flash carried even Vienna. In Virchow's own words a half century later, *"Die Krasen sind nicht wieder auf dem Markt der Wissenschaft erschienen."* The last of the *systems* of pathology had fallen.

The cellular pathology was no mere replacement, no new *system* of Virchow's own. It was the simple but early recognition of the principle to which all biological teaching had to come, cellular life. As we have seen, Schwann, following the lead of Schleiden, had proved the cellular character of organized beings, and his master Johannes Müller had ably supported their work; there remained but one step, but that the most important of all, the one that Virchow took, the recognition of the continuity of cellular life, as expressed in his immortal aphorism *"Omnis cellula e cellula."* Schwann's own concept was of a kind of repeated spontaneous generation out of a primitive body fluid, which Rokitansky accepted. This belief, with a sure clutch, Virchow throttled, making it evident for all time that one cell followed another just as surely as a man a man and a plant a plant.

He proceeded to rebuild pathology on his true conception of the human body as an organized cell state, a social system of continuous development, in which each microscopic unit performed its part. All fields of pathology were cleared by the new knowledge. Inflammation, tumor growth, degenerations, etc., were to be thought of now in their cellular relations, and in each of these fields Virchow himself led the way in bringing about the change. The physician of today can scarcely conceive how great a revolution this was. One who from his earliest student days has heard every phase of anatomy, embryology, neurology, physiology, and pathology discussed in terms of cells, can hardly picture a state of medical knowledge in which these cells had no part. We are all cellular pathologists today, taking our post-Virchovian cellular sense for granted.

In the field of degenerative changes Virchow was a pioneer. He made the original distinction between "fatty infiltration" and "fatty degeneration," and initiated the histological study of necrosis, or death of tissues. He coined the term and wrote extensively on "amyloidosis," hitherto described as "lardaceous degeneration," giving it the new name from the fact that like starch (amylum) it took on a dense coloration with iodine. In the matter of terminology he held strong opinions, insisting that "too great respect (for tradition and old terms) is a fault,

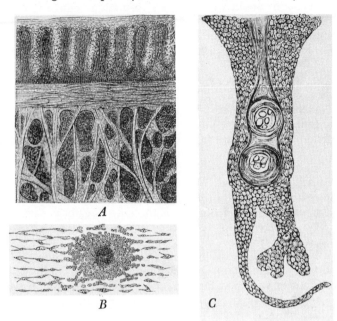

A, Carcinoma of the Uterus. *B*, a Tubercle.
C, Carcinoma of the Skin.
From the *Cellularpathologie* of Virchow, 1858

for it favors confusion." He introduced many new ones himself, including "parenchymatous inflammation," "thrombosis," "embolus," "osteoid tissue," "leukemia," and "amyloidosis."

There was never anything half-hearted about Virchow's pronouncements, so that it is not surprising that he made mistakes, and bad ones. As a matter of fact he lived to see revision or reversal of his views on inflammation, thrombophlebitis, tumors, and tuberculosis, while the advent of bacteriology ushered in a whole series of changes he could not possibly foresee. Although he wrote voluminously on tuberculosis he never made himself clear on the subject. He recognized at least two kinds, vigorously contesting the hard-gained enlightenment of the French school,

viz., (1) a post-inflammatory state, identical with the "tuberculous infiltration" described by Laënnec, and (2) the truly
tuberculous or nodular form, of which the tubercle was the
unit. On the other hand, he drew an excellent histological picture of the tubercle in the *Cellular Pathology*. The final uni-
fication brought about in after-years through recognition of the
infectious cause was a hard pill to swallow, and it is not altogether astonishing that the old fighter could never quite bring
himself to cordial terms with the great bacteriologist Robert
Koch.

The courage of his convictions led him to take a stand on the
nature of cancer and its spread, in direct contradiction to what
might have been expected in the man who discovered both the
law of continuous development of cells and embolism. Tumors,
like inflammation, always held his attention. One of his greatest
works was a monumental set of volumes on new growths, the
theory of which was germane to his cellular pathology. He
divided all neoplasms, or new growths, into two types, *homologous* and *heterologous,* the one being represented by an increase in size or number of cells of the type already present, the
other by a change in character to cells of a new type. As simple
illustrations he pointed to the common uterine "fibroid," a
benign lump in the uterus made up of muscle similar to that of
the normal organ, as an homologous change, and to cancer,
tubercle, and a variety of inflammations as heterologous change.

The more nearly benign skin tumors he considered homologous, the malignant ones heterologous, in which the essential
change, in his belief, was a conversion, or *metaplasia* as we say
today, of the underlying connective tissue. He insisted that every
cell was a direct descendant of a preëxisting cell, but saw no
difficulty in the conception of cellular transformation. Thus in
place of the blastema, Virchow in his earlier days set up connective tissue as the substrate for cancer, and an abundance of
supposed confirmation flowed to the master's hands from contemporary workers.

He had unexpected convictions on the subject of cancer
metastasis, i.e., secondary cancer growth in a new part or organ.
Not blind to the strong probability that this was an embolic
affair, he was much impressed by the fact that metastases frequently developed elsewhere than in the direct line of circulation. For example, secondary cancer nodules were commonly
found in the liver and bones and not in the lungs, when the
blood draining from the primary tumor must inevitably have

taken particulate matter straight to the latter organ. And so he stated: "The manner in which metastatic diffusion takes place seems, on the contrary, to render it probable that the transference takes place by means of certain fluids which possess the power of producing an infection disposing different parts to reproduce a mass of the same nature as the original. . . . As the salts of silver do not deposit themselves in the lungs but pass through them only to be precipitated when they reach the kidneys or the skin, so an ichorous juice may pass from a cancerous tumor through the lungs without producing any change in them, and yet at a more remote point, as for example in the bones of a far distant part, excite changes of a malignant nature."

We must not forget that in these early days of the launching of the cellular pathology Virchow had only his microscope, a fairly refined instrument by that time, razors with which he could cut moderately thin sections by hand, and the simplest of stains. He had not the advantage of the improved microtomes of later days nor the extremely helpful fixing and staining methods that are routine with us. And so it remained for Remak, Thiersch, Waldeyer, and Billroth to reconstruct Virchow's tumor pathology with omission of his errors.

Robert Remak (1815-1865), a colleague at the Charité, from the outset a clear-thinking and independent cellular pathologist, only overshadowed by Virchow, soon demonstrated by sound histological technique that skin cancers came from the epidermis and not from connective tissue. The surgeon Carl Thiersch (1822-1895) of Erlangen, without a microtome, but with good razors and an ammoniated carmine and indigo stain, prepared colored serial sections of tumors from different organs, with conclusive proof that epithelial tumors had an epithelial origin (1865). Wilhelm Waldeyer (1836-1921), a pupil of the great histologist Henle, and one of the outstanding anatomists of modern times, confirmed this source of epithelial tumors in internal organs, and turning his attention to the matter of metastasis, showed after much observation that this occurred by two routes, direct extension and embolism, both lymph and blood vessels acting as channels (1867-72). Billroth's (see page 113) wide tumor experience and direct study supported these views. The escape of certain organs from embolic metastasis, which led Virchow to give up the theory of embolism, has never been explained with complete satisfaction. The usual view, first enunciated by Cohnheim (1877), is that the "soil" is better adapted for growth in some regions than in others.

Virchow made innumerable minor contributions to pathology, for which we have not space. He was alive to every advance in biological science, although cautious in accepting all that he heard. In his own time he was reproached for refusing to accept bacteriological reports as fast as they poured in, and he opposed the Darwinian doctrine of evolution. These failings, which brought about rather bitter differences with his own pupil Edwin Klebs, and the evolutionist Ernst Haeckel (1834-1919), were after all as much the result of commendable caution as of the stubborn intolerance with which he was charged. Time and the withdrawal of many of the new germs and some of the evolutionary concepts he would not accept have justified much of his prudence.

His wide interest and indefatigable industry extended far beyond the domain of medicine. He was active in the political affairs of Germany, in which as a member of the Reichstag he took an official part. His greatest scientific interest outside of medicine was anthropology, to which he was a most fruitful contributor. Into it, which must after all have been an avocation, he carried all the zeal and conscientious thoroughness that characterized his pathology.

Physically slight, he was an awe-inspiring figure to his students. He was a hard examiner, almost cruel at times, and yet what he expected was little enough, had his candidates but known it. It was not their mistakes to which he objected; he made a great many himself. He did not expect too much detailed knowledge. He only asked evidence of independent power of observation, and a knowledge of nature's most elementary laws, i.e., some real conception of the fundamentals of biology. It was his idea that with this foundation the student could build his own structure with all its detail. And his greatest pupils fulfilled every wish. Cohnheim, Klebs, Recklinghausen, Rindfleisch, Ponfick, Orth, Hoppe-Seyler, Salkowski, and a host of others carried his ideals to brilliant heights. Through them and their pupils his influence still dominates pathology.

CHAPTER X

Pathological Histology and the Last Third of the Nineteenth Century

As we have just seen, the recognition of the cell as the unit in organized existence, by Schleiden, Müller and Schwann, laid a foundation on which Virchow rebuilt the science of pathology, which up to his time had been concerned almost solely with specific gross changes in the organs of the body. Henceforth, histological pathology and cytological or cellular pathology were to remain indispensable branches of the major science.

The impetus given by Virchow to the theory of pathology spread also to its practice. Germany, which had lagged behind France and Austria in affording recognition to the subject as a fundamental discipline in the study of biology and medicine, now began to establish full professorships in pathology throughout the country. The Würzburg and Berlin Institutes, which Virchow had built up, were soon duplicated in all the leading universities of the land. The new chairs were at first largely filled by pupils of Virchow and Rokitansky, but, developing a rapid maturity, acquired an early independence, so that soon we hear of the "Heidelberg school," the "Breslau school," etc.

The change was brought about with the minimum of upset. In a land of state control of most public enterprise it was easy to transform the hospital deadhouse to the Institute of Pathology of the university. The prosectorship of the hospital and professorship in the university became one and the same position. The new stimulus led to greatly increased frequency of post-mortem examination. Before the end of the century as many as a thousand necropsies a year were being made in the smaller university towns and five or six thousand in Berlin. With such an abundance of material the range of observation in pathological anatomy was extended enormously.

Other countries were slower to adopt this course. French pathology, which had dominated the science in the first third of the century, began to stagnate. The loss of Strasbourg in the Franco-Prussian War removed the first European chair of pathology from French control. There remained only Paris. The situation in France and Germany afforded an extraordinary contrast. French pathology was Paris pathology, while German pathology was the sum of contributions from a score of busy, productive universities.

Moreover, while hospital wards were assigned to certain professors of the Paris medical faculty, the hospitals were not actually under university control, and the necropsies were for the most part performed by internes who had no relation to the department of pathology in the university, and little intention of continuing in the subject. The chief contributions of France in the second half of the century were to be in nervous and experimental pathology.

Great Britain, in spite of its important individual contributions to the science, was even more indifferent to the merits of pathology for independent development. For many years the only chairs for the teaching of the subject were in Edinburgh and the University College of London, and strenuous effors were being made to do away with the Edinburgh position as an unwarranted academic burden and expense. In most of the medical schools, like that of Guy's Hospital, teaching and investigation in pathology remained largely in the hands of practicing physicians and surgeons, and while this emphasized in a praiseworthy way the necessity of close relationship in the teaching of pathology and medicine, the limitations imposed in time and equipment greatly held back research in new problems.

And so the main current of progress in pathology, which in the preceding century had coursed through Northern Italy, Paris, London, and Vienna, now flowed in Germany. The coincident rapid development of histology in Germany greatly favored this trend. This was largely a matter of technic. Whereas gross anatomy progressed with the aid of the scalpel and a few other familiar tools, fine anatomy soon came to require an elaborate array of apparatus and procedures for its pursuit. In the first decades of the nineteenth century, men were cutting slices of fresh tissue by hand and examining them unstained under the microscope. At the close of the century, they were hardening tissues in appropriate fluids, embedding them in rigid materials to facilitate cutting, slicing them with machinery into incredibly thin sections, and coloring them with combination stains which sharply contrasted the varying cellular elements.

This development is of such importance for the history of pathology that a few paragraphs on the history of the technic of histology are in place. This science had its beginnings in the time of Malpighi, developed slowly to the time of Bichat, when the recognition of tissue types gave it impetus, and came into its full vigor with the acceptance of the cellular doctrine of Schleiden and Schwann.

The microscope, even though Bichat ignored it, was the one essential mechanical aid. This instrument was greatly improved in the third decade of the nineteenth century, particularly through the development of the modern type of compound microscope with achromatic objectives by Joseph Jackson Lister, a London wine merchant with leisure for a scientific avocation (and the father of Lord Lister, the surgeon). Later Ernst Abbe added his well known condenser, as well as improved oculars and objectives. Many other improvements had been made in the meantime, and microscopy, instead of being a pastime, was becoming indispensable in many fields, including anatomy.

As the system of optical focussing became more sensitive, it became increasingly desirable in anatomy to have thin sections of tissue for study. With the exception of cartilage and bone, however, tissues were too soft to permit fine sectioning. Freezing was one of the first methods suggested to remedy this defect. Pieter de Riemer (1760-1831) of Holland appears to have been the pioneer in this procedure. After him most of the early microscopic anatomists made some use of it. The anatomist and surgeon Benedict Stilling (1810-1879) of Cassel used the method a great deal, particularly in his classic studies of 1843 on the histology of the central nervous system. The usual method was to immerse a container with the material to be cut in a brine freezing mixture. Succeeding improvements led to the now indispensable technic based on the rapid evaporation of ether or compressed carbonic acid gas.

Others contented themselves with freehand sections cut from tissue with razors. Knives, with two parallel blades, such as that introduced by the physiologist Gabriel Gustav Valentin (1810-1883), professor in Bern for forty-five years, were particularly useful. These were plunged or drawn rapidly through tissue with the blades screwed closely together, and thin slices secured in this way.

It was soon evident, however, that a rigid holder would be a great improvement, and mechanical microtomes were devised. The first microtome combining the two essential features of mechanical precision in movement of the knife and mechanical regulation of the object to be cut, we owe to the embryologist Wilhelm His (1831-1904) of Basel, who did his great work on the development of the chick with this instrument. This was preceded, however, by the Ranvier and other French microtomes, which were simpler and remained more popular. Before long a number of biologists in university positions invented new and improved forms, the mechanical details of which were worked out by the university technicians. One of the best of the early group, which served as a model for the most modern forms, was that devised by the German pathologist Richard Thoma, and constructed by the Heidelberg technical expert Jung (1881).

Except for frozen sections, however, the new procedure required some sort of embedding matrix to hold the tissue firmly while being cut. At first the tissue was simply placed in a slot cut in a piece of elder pith. Heidenhain introduced the use of gum arabic, and Salomon Stricker a mixture of wax and oil. To that extraordinary pioneer in many fields, Edwin Klebs, we owe the introduction of the still invaluable method of embedding in paraffin, which he described in 1869, after some years of use in his own laboratory. A decade later Mathias Duval (1844-1915) introduced the use of collodion, and shortly afterward in Germany Merkel and Schiefferdecker advocated the use of a commercial variant of collodion, celloidin, which shares with paraffin the general usage of today.

For the best embedding procedures hardening and dehydration were necessary. For the former purpose alcohol had long been in use, and it remains almost indispensable for the latter. We are indebted to Adolf Hannover (1814-1894) of Copenhagen, a pupil of Johannes Müller, for the introduction of solutions of chromic acid for fixing tissues (1844). Many modifications of the original solution were soon in use. One of the most popular was the chrom-osmium-acetic acid solution of Walther Flemming (1843-1905), the distinguished histologist whose masterly monograph on the nucleus and its division (1882) established many of our present cellular concepts, and added *Omnis nucleus e*

nucleo to Virchow's aphorism. "Zenker's fluid," containing po-
tassium bichromate and bichloride of mercury, was introduced
in 1894 by Konrad Zenker, who made claims for its usefulness
which have since been abundantly verified.

Formaldehyde solutions were first advocated in 1893 by F.
Blum, a physician of Frankfurt a. M., and his father J. Blum,
and also by F. Hermann. Within two years a large literature on
the subject had accumulated and one of the original discoverers
had occasion to lament that their priority was so soon forgotten. The substance proved of equal value in the fixation
and preservation of gross tissues, and is the essential ingredient
of several well-known solutions for this purpose, including the
very useful Kaiserling solution, which was devised in 1897
while the inventor, Carl Kaiserling, was with Virchow in Berlin.

The first important staining procedure was that of Joseph
Gerlach (1820-1896) of Mainz, who in 1847 injected the vascular
system of tissues with a transparent solution of ammoniated
carmine and gelatin. Accidentally discovering that alkaline carmine was taken up by nuclei with great avidity, he advocated
this as a nuclear stain and used it extensively in the preparation
of his *Microscopic Studies in the Field of Human Morphology*
(1858). Virchow adopted it for his work also. Alum haematoxy-
lin, the nuclear stain in most extensive use today, was first
employed by F. Böhmer of Würzburg in 1865 in the study of
tissues from a case of purulent meningitis. The discovery of
aniline dyes greatly extended staining possibilities. In the development of this field few have played as great a part as Paul
Ehrlich, who found that even living tissues could be stained
with safety by some of the dyes of this group.

Other useful procedures in tissue differentiation were the
methods of impregnation with metal salts, of which none was
more important than the silver procedure of Friedrich Daniel
von Recklinghausen (1833-1910), one of Virchow's most distinguished pupils, who was for over thirty years professor of
pathology in Strassburg. With this man we may now well begin
our consideration of the advance in pathology in the last third
of the nineteenth century. Remembered chiefly today for one
of his less important publications, the monograph (1881) which
has associated his name with the condition of multiple neuro-
fibromatosis, he left his mark in almost every field of pathology.

He was an able experimental pathologist as well as pathological anatomist. His early investigations on inflammation of
the cornea and the motility of pus corpuscles and "fixed" tissue

cells, in which the silver impregnation method and the "moist chamber," both his own inventions, were used, preceded and greatly stimulated Cohnheim, whose monumental work on inflammation will be considered in a later chapter. Recklinghausen was indeed invited to succeed Cohnheim in Leipzig, on the latter's early death.

Recklinghausen was a masterly investigator of bone pathology, his studies including fibrous or deforming osteitis, osteomalacia, rickets, and the stimulation of bone growth by certain carcinomas, the periostitis of congenital syphilis, and numerous less well-known bone diseases, between many of which he detected a relationship.

Other important studies were on thrombosis, embolism and infarction ("ball" and "hyaline" thrombi and "retrograde" embolism), hemochromatosis, which he named, various tissue degenerations, and adenomyomata of the uterus, of which he made a detailed embryological study. He and his pupils published in addition an enormous number of minor observations in pathological anatomy, and altogether made Strassburg's Institute of Pathology one of the greatest in Europe.

Other pupils of Virchow were little if any behind him. Georg Eduard Rindfleisch (1836-1908), professor in Bonn, advanced the cause of pathological histology through the publication of a valuable text on the subject. In the introduction of the book, which was dedicated to Billroth, he lamented the difficulties besetting the author of a text book of pathological histology who desired to keep pace with current discovery. "I should have good reason for complaint," he feelingly writes, "were anyone looking over this book a few years hence to forget that the views laid down in it were the views of the author in 1870."

It was indeed a crowded time. Virchow's *Archiv* was full of new discoveries. New journals were being founded. Space permits only brief mention of a few who contributed to their pages, and only those whose work expressed a major trend. The name of Edwin Klebs (1834-1913) has already been mentioned. This remarkable man, whom various vicissitudes forced to travel far, who held chairs of pathology successively in Bern, Würzburg, Prague, Zurich, and Chicago, in the seventies forged the first links between the already conventional cellular pathology and the new bacteriology. He made numerous special contributions of outstanding importance himself in the new field, which will be considered in the next chapter.

Trained originally by Virchow in the old morphological

school, he was one of the few to take open issue with his master on the fundamentals of the science. His early understanding of the parasitic nature of those diseases we now call infectious, led him to assign chief place to etiology in the study of disease, and relegate the pathological anatomy on which his teacher had labored so long and faithfully, to a secondary place. And yet he was a pathological anatomist of the highest grade himself.

An enthusiast, easily led into new and prospectively fruitful fields, he drove few of his studies to a clear-cut conclusion. But the stimulus he gave was of far-reaching effect. In bacteriology even Koch admitted his debt to Klebs. With Naunyn and Buchheim, Klebs founded and edited the *Archiv für experimentelle Pathologie und Pharmakologie* (1872), another section of the field of pathology in which he was a pioneer. His investigations on the infectious nature of endocarditis (1878) illustrate the direction of his studies.

The microbic nature of endocarditis had been made probable in 1872 by the investigation of Hjalmar Heiberg (1837-1897), professor of pathology in Christiania, a member of a famous medical family of that name, who described what appeared to him to be the mycelia of *Leptothrix* in the vegetations of a case of ulcerative endocarditis developing in a woman after childbirth. A countryman, E. Winge, had previously (1869) recorded a similar discovery under the name "mycosis endocardii." Before this, attention had several times been called to an association between vegetative endocarditis and pyemia.

Another great defection in the Virchow ranks occurred when Julius Cohnheim (1839-1884) broke with tradition on the origin of the pus cell. Once more the field of inflammation became a battleground. As Cohnheim's methods of investigation were almost entirely experimental, however, a detailed discussion of this great development will be left to the chapter on experimental pathology.

Cohnheim will always be remembered as one of the great teachers of pathology in the nineteenth century. Students flocked to Breslau, where he was professor from 1872-78, and followed him to Leipzig, when he accepted the chair in the latter university. His *Vorlesungen über allgemeine Pathologie* (1877) formed the most influential teaching compilation after Virchow's *Cellular Pathology*, and, broad as was their range, were based to a large extent on the author's own investigations.

Aside from his studies on inflammation, embolism, and infarction, which will be considered in a later chapter, Cohnheim is noted for his views on the origin of malignant growths. Impressed by the variety of congenital malformations that could be traced to accident or defect in the course of embryonic development, he conceived the idea that tumors might have a similar origin. He suggested that cells, with full capacity for orderly growth while in their normal relation to other cells, could become separated through an embryonic accident, and remain dormant in the isolated state, until in later years some stimulus activated them, whereupon growth took place with all their old-time vigor with the production of a tumor.

This theory has had great influence upon the study of malignant growth, and, while largely abandoned today in its general applications, has proved highly fertile in the understanding of teratomas. The well-known theory of Hugo Ribbert (1855-1920) of Bonn may be considered a modification of the Cohnheim view. Ribbert likewise believed that tumors might develop from isolated cells which retained a capacity for individual growth, but attributed the isolation not to embryonic accident, but to a separation of a group of cells from their normal relations in adult life, as a result of irregular growth of other tissues. These cells, he suggested, normal in their accustomed relations, might grow abnormally in the new environment.

The tendency of certain types of malignant growth to occur late in life was explained by Ribbert, as previously by Thiersch and Waldeyer, on the basis of a disturbed balance of tissue equilibrium permitting one tissue to overgrow another. These theories, stimulating as they have proved to investigation, have ultimately proved inadequate to cover all the facts.

Cohnheim's most distinguished pupil was Carl Weigert (1845-1904), who opened the way for an understanding of the major facts of tissue degeneration and necrosis. He was born in the small town of Münsterberg, Silesia. Before his association with Cohnheim he came under the stimulating influence of Virchow, Heidenhain, Lebert, and Waldeyer. After a short service as army surgeon in the Franco-Prussian War he entered the Breslau medical clinic. Here he took advantage of an opportunity to make an intensive microscopic study of the skin eruption of smallpox. This investigation laid the ground for his great work on coagulation necrosis and brought him to the attention of Cohnheim, who took him as assistant. Thereafter he remained with the great experimental pathologist, following him to Leipzig as *extraordinarius,* supplementing the brilliant experiments of his chief with equally able achievement in the field of mor-

phology. He suffered keen disappointment in not being invited
to succeed Cohnheim at Leipzig, at the latter's death in 1884.
Apparently as a Jew he was not acceptable; his qualifications
for the position were beyond question and openly admitted. He
moved to Frankfurt a. M., where he remained nearly twenty
years in active research. He died suddenly in the midst of his
labors, at the age of fifty-nine, of coronary thrombosis.

The smallpox epidemic of 1871-72, occurring while he was an
assistant in medicine in Breslau, started his career in two important fields. An early student of the part played by bacteria in
contagious disease and at the same time an expert in the technic
of histology, he was led to employ the staining methods of the
latter in the search for bacteria. He used the nuclear dye carmine, and the first successful staining of bacteria in tissues
rewarded his efforts. Although the germs discovered proved to
have only a secondary relation to smallpox, the event was outstanding as a landmark in bacteriology, as it facilitated further
research enormously.

In the course of the same smallpox study he was impressed
by the highly destructive but sharply circumscribed effect of
the unknown smallpox virus upon the affected skin. Later studies
on diphtheria supported his early views. For his excellent picture of the state of the tissue in these lesions, and the process
concerned in their development, Cohnheim coined the term
"coagulation necrosis." Mature investigation led Weigert to
consider the anemic infarct as the prototype of coagulation
necrosis, "which could not occur unless the tissue itself possessed
a coagulable substance, and died in such a way that it could
still be permeated by a coagulable plasmatic fluid, without any
fermentative change or suppurative process intervening to prevent the process." Embolism and infarction occupied much of
his attention; he was the first to describe accurately infarction
of the heart (1880).

His studies on degeneration of tissues carried him to the
problems of repair, particularly in connection with chronic
nephritis, cirrhosis of the liver, and fibrosis of the myocardium.
He concluded that whenever epithelium or analogous tissue was
destroyed, an overgrowth of interstitial connective tissue took
place, provided suppuration did not occur and the interstitial
tissue itself was not totally destroyed. This belief in growth as a
sequel of loss of other tissue was opposed to the view of Virchow, who taught that cell growth took place only as a result of
a direct stimulus. Weigert's emphasis on the primary excess in

new production of tissue in repair formed the basis of the celebrated side-chain theory of immunity developed later by Weigert's cousin Paul Ehrlich.

Weigert was a masterly technician. His development of the method of serial sections of tissue, and elaboration of special stains, were as fruitful for general histology and neurology as for pathology. Of his many other investigations probably the outstanding was his work on miliary tuberculosis (1877-86), in which he called attention to tubercles within the walls of veins as the source of dissemination of the virus of the disease.

Of the same period was Ernst Ziegler (1849-1905), Swiss-born, a student of Klebs and Rindfleisch, who spent the best part of his life as professor of pathology in Freiburg, and who influenced the science profoundly through his accomplishments in its organization, as well as by specific contributions. A large share of the leading pathologists all over the world a generation ago were brought up on Ziegler's great *Text of General Pathology and Pathological Anatomy,* first published in 1881, which has appeared in many editions and translations and is still one of the leading works on the subject. He founded and edited two journals, which have been second in influence only to Virchow's *Archiv,* the *Beiträge zur pathologischen Anatomie und allgemeinen Pathologie* (1886, "Ziegler's *Beiträge*") and the *Centralblatt für allgemeine Pathologie und pathologische Anatomie* (1890). As an investigator he was concerned chiefly with the causes of disease, and with inflammation, inflammatory new growth, and repair, in other words the protective forces of the body.

Of the rest who took part in the great development of German pathology only a few can be mentioned in this brief account. Friedrich Albert von Zenker (1825-1898), professor in Dresden (1855-62) and Erlangen (1862-95), is remembered chiefly for his monograph on waxy degeneration of certain voluntary muscles in typhoid fever. He made important contributions also on trichinosis, dust inhalation, and fat embolism, which he was one of the first to describe (1862). Ernst Neumann (1834-1918) of Königsberg, in the course of his long and active life, made many important observations on the subject of regeneration of tissues after injury. His important pioneer investigations on the bone-marrow greatly improved the understanding of the leukemias. Julius Arnold (1835-1915) made Heidelberg one of the outstanding schools of pathology in Germany. His

PLATE XXXVI

PLATE XXXVII

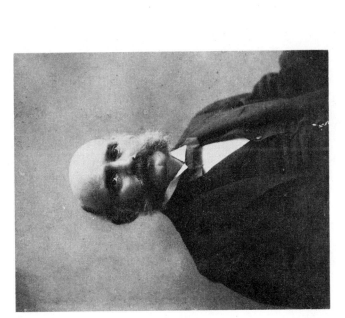

CARL WEIGERT (1845-1904)

MICROSCOPIC SECTIONS OF SMALLPOX PUSTULES
From Weigert's *Die Pocken-Effloreszenzen*, 1874

PLATE XXXVIII

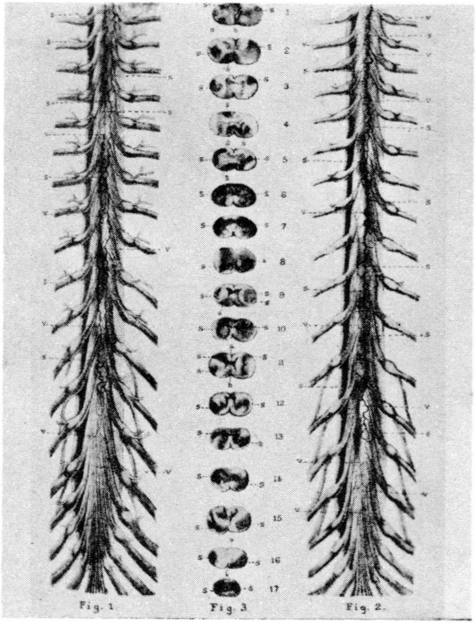

DISSEMINATED SCLEROSIS OF THE SPINAL CORD
From Charcot's *Diseases of the Nervous System*
1872-93

PLATE XXXIX

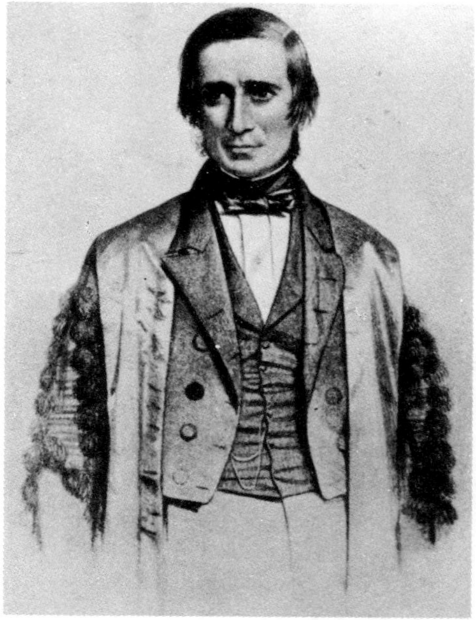

SIR JAMES PAGET (1814-1899)
Courtesy of Longmans, Green and Company

own studies on nuclear and cell division, on the fine anatomy of the miliary tubercle (1880-82), and on the effects caused by inhalation of dust and metal particles (1885-90) were particularly important.

Another distinguished, long-lived pathologist was Karl Joseph Eberth (1835-1926) of Zurich, whose experiments on thrombosis (1885-86), partly carried out with his pupil Schimmelbusch, brought out the importance of stagnation of the blood flow and the rôle played by the blood platelets in coagulation, confirming previous statements on the platelets by Giulio Bizzozero of Turin (1882) and the Paris clinician and hematologist Georges Hayem (1882). Eberth is perhaps still better known as the discoverer of the typhoid bacillus (1880). Emil Ponfick (1844-1913), a student of Recklinghausen and Virchow, is especially notable for establishing the pathological nature of human actinomycosis (1880), the parasite of which had been well studied previously, particularly by Otto Bollinger (1876) and Oscar Israel (1878). The disease had once been thought a malignant tumor. Richard Thoma, a life-long student of diseases of arteries, furnished pathology with one of its most nearly satisfying explanations of arteriosclerosis, based on the analogy of the physiological postnatal sclerosis of the vessels to the placenta. The conception of thickening of the arterial intima as a compensation for weakening of the media forms the essence of his theory. Thoma is known also for his technical improvements in the apparatus for blood counting and section cutting. Johannes Orth (1847-1923) succeeded Virchow in 1902 in the chair of pathology in Berlin, and editorship of Virchow's *Archiv*.

In the meantime, except in one field, French pathological anatomy had stagnated. This domain was neuropathology and its leader was Jean-Martin Charcot (1825-1893), who conducted at the Salpêtrière in Paris the greatest of the modern neurological clinics. Trained in the old Paris school of pathological anatomy and for a time himself incumbent of the chair in this subject, he carried the pathological point of view into neurology, going far in the explanation of many puzzling clinical pictures in this difficult field. One of his most notable achievements was the anatomical elucidation of the symptoms dependent on multiple sclerosis, the first anatomical descriptions of which he credited to Cruveilhier and Carswell. He made accurate histological studies of the spinal cord in locomotor ataxia, giving credit for the original description to Hutin (1827), and frankly claiming the whole subject as a "French conquest," and "part of the great anatomo-pathological epoch inaugurated by Laënnec." Charcot himself described the lesion and explained the symptom complex of amyotrophic lateral sclerosis. The joint affections occurring in certain diseases of the central system are still known as "Charcot joints."

Charcot and Victor Cornil first demonstrated the atrophy of the anterior horns of the spinal cord in infantile paralysis, a discovery which Duchenne (1806-1875) had predicted. Vulpian and Prévost pointed out the lesion in the motor nerve cells shortly afterward (1866). A masterly and comprehensive study of diseases of the spinal cord was made by Vulpian's pupil, Jules Déjerine (1849-1917), a Swiss-born Frenchman who developed an early interest in neuropathology and ultimately succeeded to the chair first occupied by Charcot in the Salpêtrière. He is especially notable for his localization of brain lesions in the various types of aphasia. His achievements were the outcome of the most painstaking histological examination of the degenerated regions. The results of Déjerine and others of the Charcot school served to correct false inferences in cerebral localization that had been accumulating since the time of Willis from unwarranted application of results in laboratory animals to man.

Charcot's ablest pupil was Pierre Marie, who described acromegaly in 1886 and later called attention to the relation of the hypophysis to this disease, basing his conclusion as much on the post-mortem discoveries of others as on his own. As a matter of fact, an association between gigantism and pituitary enlargement had been repeatedly noted. Among those reporting the coincidence was the pathologist Edwin Klebs, who published in 1884, in collaboration with the clinician Fritsche, a full account of a case in which gigantic stature, with especially marked enlargement of the skull, and increase in size of the hypophysis were conspicuous features. A large persisting thymus in the same patient, however, left the authors confused, and so it remained for others to establish the etiological association with the hypophysis.

Marie's name is still given to that condition known as hypertrophic osteo-arthropathy, following his original description in 1890. As a faithful disciple of Charcot, he pursued his teacher's trend in the pathology of the central nervous system. It is significant that Marie achieved eminence in both neuropathology and the study of physiological abnormalities of the ductless glands. Both fields were largely under French domination. The two leaders in the latter science, both likewise distinguished in the former, were Claude Bernard and Charles-Édouard Brown-Séquard. As their work was largely experimental, its consideration will be left to a later chapter.

The leading French histologist of the period, Charles-Philippe Robin (1821-1885), through his investigations of the fine anatomy of the central nervous system played an important part in the great French neurological development. He was also the founder, with Charcot, of the important *Journal de l'Anatomie et de la Physiologie Normales et Pathologiques de l'Homme et des Animaux* (1864).

The state of English pathology has already been indicated. The teaching and development of the subject were in the hands of able but busy practicing physicians and surgeons. Clinicians in both fields made a number of contributions of major importance, however. The work of Sir William Gull (1816-1890), who was associated with Guy's Hospital all his professional life, rivaled that of the leaders in the French school in neuropathology. His was among the first good descriptions of the spinal lesion of locomotor ataxia, or tabes dorsalis, and he left an excellent account of aneurysms of the cerebral arteries. His greatest work, however, was probably his study, in conjunction with Henry G. Sutton, of "arterio-capillary fibrosis" in chronic nephritis, which appeared in 1872. This is the first clear description of arteriolo-sclerotic atrophy of the kidney, and while Gull and his associate did not make the distinction between chronic nephritis and the arteriolo-sclerotic kidney that is made today, they emphasized quite correctly the association of the atrophied kidney with generalized thickening of the arterioles, which they introduced as a special variety of the well known arteriosclerosis.

At the rival hospital and school of St. Bartholomew the surgeon Sir James Paget (1814-1899) greatly stimulated surgical pathology. His *Lectures on Tumors* appeared in 1851 and his great *Surgical Pathology* in 1863. An infected dissection wound which incapacitated him for three months in 1871 inspired him to write a lecture and monograph on *Dissection Poisons*. Two diseases are named after Paget, in recognition of his original descriptions, eczema of the nipple with cancer (1874) and osteitis deformans (1877-82).

Two other surgeons deserve mention for their stimulus to surgical pathology, Sir Benjamin Brodie (1783-1862), who made important observations on diseases of the bones and joints, and Sir Jonathan Hutchinson (1828-1913), who is especially to be remembered for his work on the stigmata of congenital syphilis (the chronic inflammation of the cornea, the notched incisor teeth and disease of the internal ear, commonly grouped as "Hutchinson's triad").

In America pathology was just getting under way. Much of the early development of medical science in this country centered about the University of Pennsylvania, where under the provostship of William Pepper (1843-1898) many precedents in American medical education were established. Pepper edited a pioneer large American *System of Medicine* (1886). He is notable in pathology for the first description of the changes in the bone-marrow in pernicious anemia (1875). This disease had been vaguely recognized since Addison's description in 1855. Biermer of Zurich redescribed it in 1872. Cohnheim in studying the tissues from a case of Biermer's in 1876 noted the bone-marrow changes, unaware of Pepper's prior description. Pepper, much impressed by the work of Neumann, Waldeyer, and Ponfick on the leukemias and Cohnheim's separation of the condition of pseudoleukemia (1865), concluded in his able article on pernicious anemia that "an affection of the chief blood-making tissues, spleen, lymphatic glands and marrow of the bones" was at the basis of all of them.

The first important American textbook of pathology after that of Samuel Gross emanated from the hands of Francis Delafield (1841-1915), Professor of the Practice of Medicine in the College of Physicians and Surgeons of Columbia University in New York, and T. Mitchell Prudden (1849-1924), Professor of Pathology in the same institution. It has passed through many editions since its first appearance in 1885.

Still more influential in American pathology have been Sir William Osler (1849-1919) and William Henry Welch (1850-1934). The first, Canadian born and educated, brought the best English scholarly tradition to American medicine and an extraordinary teaching ability. At McGill, Pennsylvania, and Johns Hopkins Universities he was the outstanding teacher of internal medicine in the New World. He was keenly appreciative of the fundamental importance of an understanding of pathology for progress in medicine, and made many minor contributions in the subject himself. William Welch was long held and revered as the dean of American pathology. His chief accomplishments were in the experimental pathology which will be treated in a later chapter.

We shall now consider a spectacular development which strongly bent the course of pathological research, the rise of bacteriology, which took place coincidently with the events described in this chapter.

CHAPTER XI

The Rise of Bacteriology and Immunology

The last quarter of the nineteenth century proved extra-ordinarily rich for the development of pathology, not only through the extension of pathological histology and the closer approach of physiology and pathology through experiment, but particularly through remarkable discoveries on the cause of disease. The new science of bacteriology solved some of the major problems which had puzzled medicine for twenty centuries.

The idea of contagion was no new one. Definite notions had existed on it since ancient times. The contagious element of the plague and syphilis was too evident to be missed. Medical beliefs on the former had found far-reaching expression in the lay writings of Boccaccio (1358) and Defoe (1722). Fracastoro's great book on contagion and his special studies on syphilis, with the hundreds of later writings on this subject, defined the element of contagion in its spread clearly. Leprosy, an endemic scourge from the twelfth to the fourteenth centuries, was considered transferable and the effectiveness of quarantine measures bore out the belief. Contagion was indeed credited to a living virus, and speculation on this *contagium animatum* was extended to investigation, Athanasius Kircher and Antonj van Leeuwenhoek (see Chapter IV) in their search with feeble microscopes actually discovering subvisible living things.

The early years of the eighteenth century were particularly notable for expressions on the specificity of contagious diseases and suggestions as to the mode of their transmission. A pioneer in the doctrine of specific contagion and immunity, the English country physician Thomas Fuller (1654-1734) laid down his views in the following striking way: "The Pestilence can never breed the Small-Pox, nor the Small-Pox the Measles, nor they the Crystals or Chicken-Pox, any more than a Hen can breed a Duck, a Wolf a Sheep, or a Thistle Figs; and consequently one Sort cannot be a Preservative against any other Sort."

The concept of immunity is likewise old. The ancients recognized that one seizure with certain diseases afforded protection against subsequent attacks. Centuries ago, the Chinese put this knowledge into practice by deliberately passing smallpox from person to person by inoculation of the pustular material, the disease so produced proving mild but immunizing against later natural contagion. This procedure of "variolation" was in later times widely practiced throughout the civilized world.

The real foundations of immunology came with the introduction of *vaccination* by Edward Jenner (1749-1823), an English physician and one of John Hunter's most distinguished pupils, who developed a far safer, but equally effective method of immunization against smallpox. The statement of a dairymaid, "I cannot take the smallpox because I have had the cowpox," expressing the current rural English view, impelled him to make a direct test of its correctness. In May 1796 he transferred matter from a cowpox lesion on the arm of a milkmaid to a healthy boy, and in July followed it up with genuine smallpox virus. The boy failed to develop the latter disease.

This preliminary success in causing a harmless lesion to protect against the similar, but vastly more serious smallpox justified repetition on a grand scale. His first twenty-three cases were published in 1798, the method being designated "vaccination" in reference to the source (*vacca,* cow) of the injected material. Immediate recognition of the method's worth led to wholesale vaccination in Europe and America, and within a short space of time smallpox, once an almost universal disease, became a rarity in all civilized communities. No other prophylactic measure in medicine has ever been attended by the same degree of success, if we except the insistence of Holmes and Semmelweis (page 112) on simple cleanliness in childbirth.

Jenner's triumph, no less than the success of quarantine in leprosy and plague, was the result of empirical observation and deduction. Further scientific progress in the control of contagion demanded instruments and methods not available in Jenner's time. Only with improvement of the microscope was such progress possible, and without the chemical assistance of synthetic stains even the microscope was a feeble tool.

The finding of microbes merely kept pace with the development of these facilities, the larger microscopic parasites being discovered first and the smaller bacteria only much later. Shortly after the notable development of acromatic lenses between 1810 and 1830, the larger parasites began to be discovered. In 1839 the Berlin clinician Johann Lukas Schönlein (1793-1864) found the cause of favus. In 1842 his assistant Remak reproduced the disease in himself with Schönlein's organism. Other skin parasites were detected shortly afterwards, and the fungi now connected with aspergillosis and actinomycosis were discovered about the same time. In the meantime, the Italian physician Agostino Bassi (1773-1856) had clearly shown the causal relation of certain microörganisms to the muscardine disease of silkworms (1837), and prophesied the discovery of microbes of animal or vegetable origin as causal agents of smallpox, plague, syphilis, and other human diseases.

The importance of Bassi's work was immediately recognized in Germany by Henle, and grasped in many other quarters likewise. In fact suggestions on microbic contagion in disease began to pour in so fast that Henle, although predicting that microbiology was to throw etiological light into many of the obscurities of pathology, felt impelled to draw certain limitations on the gathering mass of speculation. In his famous essay *On Miasms and Contagion* (1840), he laid down postulates on the etiological relation of microbes to disease, which were later extended by Koch as the fundamental principles of bacteriology. Henle insisted in a general way on (1) demonstration of constancy in the association of a given disease and its supposed parasitic cause, as well as its absence in other diseases, (2) isolation and separation from other microbes, and finally, (3) proof of the power of the isolated germ to produce disease, and did much to curb the reckless exploitation of newly discovered germs already under way.

It was not long afterward that most of these demands were satisfied for one disease by Casimir Davaine, who, after discovering and recording the presence of peculiar minute rods in the blood of a sheep dead of anthrax somewhat indifferently in 1850, returned to the subject with great vigor in 1863 after Pasteur's views on microbic fermentation had been published. Davaine soon showed that the disease was transferable from a sick animal to a well by inoculation of the former's blood, even diluted a million times, while not transmissible with blood from another well animal containing none of the rodlets he had

PLATE XL

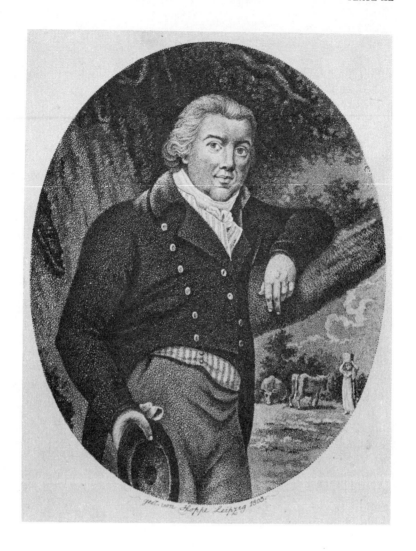

EDWARD JENNER (1749-1823)

PLATE XLI

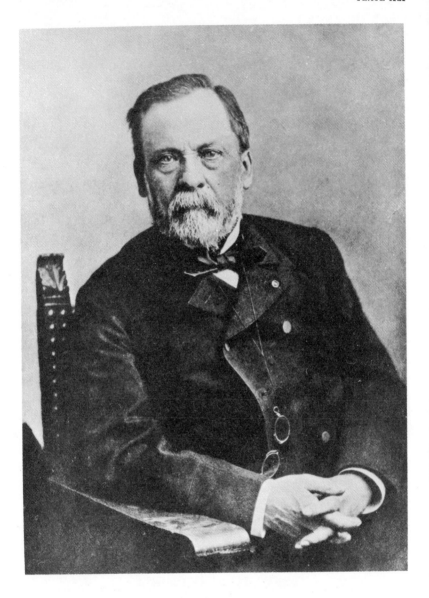

LOUIS PASTEUR (1822-1895)
Courtesy of National Library of Medicine

described. The anthrax microörganism, one of the largest of bacteria, was to prove useful several times in giving bacteriology its start, both Pasteur and Koch publishing important works on it.

From these two men the study of infection derived its greatest impetus, and it is a noteworthy fact that the first of them to enter the field was neither a physician nor a skilled biologist, but a man with the best of training in a quite different science, chemistry. Louis Pasteur (1822-1895), born in the small town of Dôle in the department of Jura, took up the latter study in his preparatory training and made it his major interest in the École Normale in Paris, from which he graduated in 1847.

The year after his graduation, while serving as professor of physics in Dijon, he made the discovery that formed the starting point for all his later brilliant studies in bacteriology, viz., that by means of fermentation he could separate the two varieties of tartaric acid distinguished by their capacity to rotate the plane of polarized light in opposite directions. He had himself already separated these types on a crystallographic basis. One form, he found, was destroyed by fermentation, the other not. This discovery opened the way for a more exact understanding of the essential nature of ferment action.

From this he developed an intense interest in the subject of fermentation in general, out of which grew his system of controlling undesired fermentation in beer and wine, which proved of tremendous industrial importance for France. Our term "pasteurization" dates from these studies. His studies on the microbic cause of the *pébrine,* a new silkworm disease in the south of France, and advocation of suitable quarantine measures in the shipping and use of seed had already proved of equal value to his country.

At the same time, he was conducting masterly investigations on spontaneous generation. This was an old subject of scientific quarrel. In 1668 the Italian physician and naturalist Francesco Redi (1626-1697) had for a time silenced believers in the spontaneous origin of grubs and maggots in decaying meat by showing that flies brought the eggs for their development. New evidence, however, was constantly being presented for spontaneous birth of animalcules in putrefying matter. Another Italian, an able physiologist, Lazaro Spallanzani (1729-1799), overthrew the rising doctrine of a primitive vegetative force giving rise to living forms. Even the philosopher Voltaire took a hand in the struggle, with sarcastic flings at the spontaneous generationists. But the belief would not down. Theodor Schwann, the founder of the teaching of animal cells, opposed the theory by showing, like Spallanzani, that proper heating of organic matter prevented its putrefaction (1836).

Nevertheless, in 1860 the problem was as much alive as ever. As Pasteur became more deeply engaged in the study of fermentation, the question grew more and more insistent, until it became obvious that it must be settled before his results on specificity in type of fermentation could have any significance. In a remarkable piece of work in the early sixties he overcame all opposition and truly cleared the ground for a science of bacteriology. The methods evolved for maintaining the sterility of fluids in his experiments were to prove as important for the technic of the science as the results were for its theory.

All these studies inevitably led Pasteur into the study of infectious disease. He extended his views on fermentation to the subject of putrefaction and attracted the attention of the British surgeon, Joseph Lister (1827-1912). As late as 1870 copious suppuration of wounds, if not actually promoted with filth as in former days, was still considered a desirable event. Lister soon showed that measures to prevent the development of microbes in wounds and surgical procedures in general prevented suppuration and likewise permitted healing by first intention with a minimum of scarring and distress and danger to the life of the patient. From this start came our modern aseptic surgery.

Specificity in microbic cause of disease was the logical extension of Pasteur's ideas on specificity in type of fermentation. Exposure to one kind of disease, he said, is not followed by the outbreak of a different kind of disease, any more than sowing of beer with the germs he had found responsible for a given type of beer "disease" was followed by some other disease. No one man could carry his ideas far without help in such a huge field, but Pasteur had the aid of a brilliant series of associates, and with their help bacteria in septic processes were soon found.

Of greater importance, however, than the mere discovery and isolation of bacteria was his specific immunization in anthrax and chicken cholera, by inoculating cattle and fowl respectively with heated, dried, or otherwise "attenuated" microörganisms of the disease. His greatest success was in rabies, for which he determined the seat of the infection and therefore source of immunizing material, without being able, however, to detect the offending germ. The various Pasteur Institutes scattered over the world, together with the brilliant line of personal pupils in charge of many of them, are the greatest monument to Pasteur's memory.

Thus, through the life work of the Frenchman Pasteur came much of the early theory of bacteriology and immunology. The practice developed even more extensively in the hands of the great German Robert Koch (1843-1910), a native of Hannover and a graduate of Göttingen in 1866, where, as we have seen, Jacob Henle was professor of anatomy. Henle's advanced views on bacteriology, summarized a few pages back, must have profoundly influenced Koch. After his graduation Koch entered upon the practice of medicine, but maintained his special interest in microbes and their effects. His first studies were on the life history and infecting power of the germ of anthrax. In a magnificent piece of work he isolated the tiny rod that Davaine and others had seen, and after many successive generations in artificial culture outside the animal body was still able to reproduce the disease by injecting the culture into animals. Before publishing his results he submitted them to a man already distinguished for his studies on the bacteria of plants, the influential director of the Botanical Institute of Breslau, Ferdinand Cohn (1828-1898), who promptly invited Koch to demonstrate his work. The demonstration before the brilliant Breslau group marked an epoch in bacteriology. It made a profound impression on Cohnheim and Weigert, whose work was to fit in with Koch's in later years in extraordinary fashion.

Koch's service in the understanding of the bacteriology of disease was threefold. He developed methods for discovering bacteria and isolating them in pure culture free from all other forms; he defined the conditions for recognizing a particular germ as the cause of a particular disease; and finally, he made a series of brilliant discoveries of specific disease-producing bacteria himself.

In the first of these he used methods put forth by Carl Weigert (1845-1904), who was the first to stain bacteria in tissues. In 1871, in his studies on smallpox, Weigert, as we have seen, had stained the bacteria now known to be simply secondary invaders in the pustules of the disease with the animal dye carmine, obtained from cochineal. In 1875, when aniline dye chemistry had made enormous progress in Germany, Weigert, in studying ulceration around the umbilical cord in a newborn child, found little granular masses in the pus, which proved to be bacteria, and stained beautifully with the new aniline dye, methyl violet.

Koch found that nearly all bacteria could be fixed to a glass slide by heat and readily stained with these new dyes.

Still more fruitful were Koch's methods for isolating pure strains of bacteria. These were described in 1881 after a monumental work on *Wound Infection* had established his place as the coming bacteriologist of Germany, and Cohnheim and others, in recognition of the event, had secured his appointment in the Imperial Health Department in Berlin. Koch had previously used liquid meat infusions in his cultivation of microörganisms, but it was difficult to separate different kinds from one another when all grew equally well in this nutritive medium. A clever method solved this problem. He supplemented the meat extract with gelatine in the warm, added his mixture of bacteria, mixed them thoroughly in the liquid mass, and then allowed the latter to cool and turn solid. In the course of the next day or two the different and now widely separated bacteria developed into individual colonies, each a pure strain capable of being removed in part from the "gelatine plate" and grown indefinitely in new media without further admixture with other microörganisms.

Koch's work on wound infection had established the sharp specificity of bacteria found in septic and purulent processes, and his later work fortified this by demonstrating their capacity to breed true in all subsequent generations. In the year following his development of special isolation methods, he made his great discovery of the cause of tuberculosis. As we have seen in preceding chapters, the varying manifestations of this disease had been a stumbling block to physicians since the earliest times. Laënnec had finally reduced consumption to the rank of a single disease, and had gone on record against the prevalent view that it might be the sequel of a variety of inflammations. Virchow, the commanding figure of a later day, reversed this view, distinguishing two broad types of tuberculosis and tracing one of them to previous inflammation. Another Frenchman, Jean-Antoine Villemin (1827-1892), however, soon brought forth the startling proof that tuberculosis could be transmitted from man to animals, and from animal to animal indefinitely, by simply injecting some of the material from the lesions into the normal animal. This proof, overwhelming as it was, failed of acceptance until Virchow's own pupil Julius Cohnheim (1839-1884) placed the matter beyond doubt by inoculating tuberculous material into the anterior chamber of a rabbit's eye, where the development of the lesion could be watched from day to day.

Koch completed the story by discovering the inciting micro-

PLATE XLIII

PLATE XLII

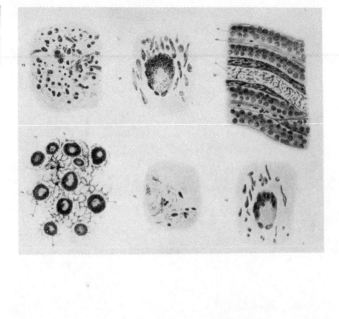

TUBERCULOUS LESIONS WITH TUBERCLE BACILLI
From Koch's *Ätiologie der Tuberkulose*, 1882

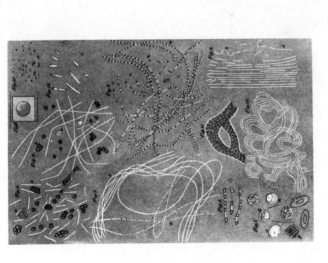

ANTHRAX BACILLI
From Koch's *Ätiologie der Milzbrandkrankheit*, 1876

PLATE XLIV

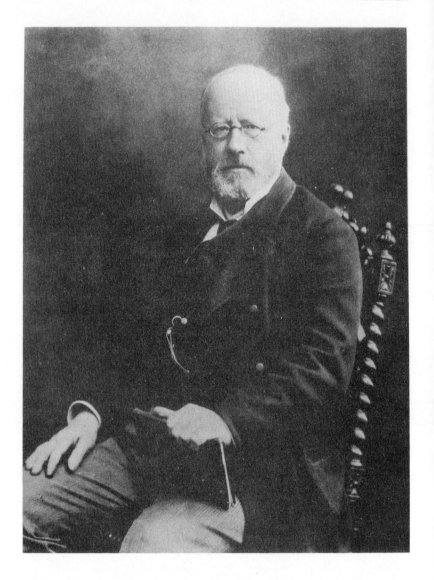

EDWIN KLEBS (1834-1913)
Reproduced through the courtesy of Lt. Col. Fielding H.
Garrison

örganism, which had escaped his predecessors in the field, through a combination of patience and ingenious technic. In publishing his results he laid down the laws since considered fundamental to the science, viz., that before recognition as the cause of a disease a germ (1) must be found constantly associated with that disease, (2) must be isolated from a lesion of that disease apart from other germs, (3) must reproduce the disease in a suitable animal on inoculation in pure culture, and finally (4) be found again in the lesions of this artificially produced disease.

Every year now was bringing a fresh triumph. In 1883, in the Orient as the head of the German Cholera Commission, he discovered the cholera vibrio, thereby providing a ready and successful means of quarantine control of this disease. Less important but still notable discoveries continued to fill the remaining years of his life. He came to occupy about the same position in bacteriology as Virchow in pathology, both men being recipients of the highest state recognition in their own country and international fame in their respective branches of science. Koch's pupils continued his brilliant achievements just as Virchow's carried on the cellular pathology.

It was another man, and something of a rival of both, however, who did the most in the early days of bacteriology to align the new science with pathology. This was Edwin Klebs (1834-1913), to whose versatility in pathology attention has already been drawn. Few of the important diseases now recognized as infectious escaped his early attention. He stands with Koch and Billroth as one of the first to investigate the relation of bacteria to wound sepsis. Scarcely behind Pasteur and Chamberland, he was one of the first to sterilize fluids by filtration. He preceded Koch in attempting the use of solid cultures for bacteria. He seems to have had a peculiar genius for opening the way in every department and leaving the field for someone else to win the major credit. He was an early and almost successful investigator of the bacterial cause of typhoid fever and tuberculosis, but it is only in connection with diphtheria, the causal agent of which is often called the "Klebs-Löffler bacillus," that his investigations were pushed to a clear-cut conclusion. He was a pioneer in the experimental transmission of infectious disease by feeding. He left many errors on record, but his tremendous industry and experimental fertility proved an enormous stimulus to others in the field.

The next to the last decade of the nineteenth century brought in the discoveries of most of the specific bacteria of infectious disease. The tools and the methods were at last at hand. Activity was feverish. The germs of all diseases were going to be found, and the find was to be followed by the cure. Disease, barring a few unavoidable degenerations to which the flesh inevitably seemed heir, was to be wiped out. The millennium seemed at hand.

The pupils and assistants of Koch played a great part in the work. Friedrich Löffler (1852-1915), one of them, shared with Klebs the discovery of the diphtheria bacillus, and added the bacillus of glanders to the growing list. Another chapter was furnished in the long history of typhoid fever when Karl Joseph Eberth (1835-1926) described the typhoid bacillus in 1880 and Georg Gaffky (1850-1918), another of Koch's associates, isolated it in pure culture in 1884.

The peculiar microscopic rod in leprous lesions, seen and described by the Norwegian Armauer Hansen (1841-1912) in 1871, was classed in the group of bacteria by the Berlin bacteriologist and specialist in venereal diseases Albert Neisser (1855-1916) in 1879, the same year that Neisser discovered the gonococcus in gonorrhoeal pus. The pneumococcus, now known to exist in several types, was seen early and often. Pasteur, George Miller Sternberg (1838-1915), Surgeon General of the United States Army, and Albert Fränkel (1848-1916) in Germany share the credit for its earliest descriptions. Klebs, as usual, had apparently seen it before any of them, while Anton Weichselbaum (1845-1920) left one of the best descriptions. Weichselbaum, fourth incumbent in the professorship of pathological anatomy in the Rokitansky line in Vienna, is chiefly remembered in bacteriology for his discovery of the meningococcus of acute cerebrospinal fever in 1887.

The bacillus responsible for tetanus was discovered by Arthur Nicolaier in Göttingen in 1884, shortly after the Italians Carlo and Rattone had proved the infective character of the disease, and first grown in pure culture in 1885 by the able, German-trained Japanese bacteriologist Shibasaburo Kitasato. Kitasato and Alexandre Yersin simultaneously and independently discovered the cause of bubonic plague in the course of the great epidemic which began in Hong Kong in 1894, thus bringing to earth the long-sought cause of another of the oldest and best known diseases of mankind. Another Japanese, K. Shiga, in searching stools for the amoebae shortly before established as the cause of tropical dysentery by Koch and Kartulis in Egypt and Osler and his associates in America, failed to find them, but isolated from the Japanese type of dysentery the bacillus which has since gone by his name. In 1900 Simon Flexner isolated a different species of dysentery bacillus. Many shared in the early descriptions of the staphylococcus and streptococcus, the commonest invaders in the wound infections.

Most amazingly, it was left to the twentieth century to discover the cause of syphilis, which had been one of the mainstays of the theories of a *contagium animatum* since Fracastoro's early publications. Cause after cause bobbed up in the hands of eager young bacteriologists, only to be discarded a month later. In 1905 the dermatologist Lassar collected one hundred and twenty-five causes reported in the preceding twenty-five years, but in the same year the protozoölogist Fritz Schaudinn (1871-1906) and Erich Hoffmann, with better technic than their predecessors, discovered the true cause, the spirochaeta pallida.

In the meantime, the sciences of immunology and protective immunization had made tremendous strides. Their progress brought in first another recrudescence of humoral pathology, next a conflicting solidist pathology, and finally a clear, and perhaps lasting reconciliation of the two. The new humoral pathology developed in the recognition of specific bacterial toxins and antitoxins. Two of Pasteur's pupils, Émile Roux and Alexandre Yersin, in 1888 had discovered poisonous properties in nutritive broth that had served for the cultivation of diphtheria bacilli. Almost at the same time, Kitasato showed that cultures of the tetanus bacillus, which he had himself isolated, were still highly toxic for animals after all the bacilli had been removed by filtration. In this case too a specific poison had appeared in the medium of growth. Two years later in Koch's Institute Emil von Behring (1854-1817), with Kitasato, showed that the blood serum of animals injected with this poison after a time developed the capacity to neutralize it so that amounts ordinarily fatal could now be injected with impunity. Moreover if removed from the immunized animal and injected into another animal this serum could protect that one likewise against the toxin.

For a few eager months it seemed as if infectious disease was to be conquered through the use of specific antitoxins. Simultaneously with tetanus antitoxin came diphtheria antitoxin, developed by Behring and associates. Small laboratory experiments were soon followed by a world-wide confirmation in man, and a sharp drop occurred in the diphtheria rate in all countries. This success ranks as one of the most brilliant of all achievements in the treatment of disease. It soon became sadly apparent, however, that the original hopes were over-optimistic, for the antitoxin treatment was found applicable to only a relatively small number of the infectious diseases.

A humoral defense was soon recognized, however, not only against the poisons of bacteria but against the germs themselves. Hans Buchner in 1889 had explained the resistance of blood to putrefaction, that character which had so impressed John Hunter, by demonstrating its innate capacity to kill bacteria. In 1894 Richard Pfeiffer found that cholera vibrios injected into the peritoneal cavity of a guinea pig immunized against the same organism, quickly lost their motility, became granular, and finally went to pieces. Similar dissolution did not follow the introduction of the cholera vibrio into a normal animal. The immune animal's serum had acquired a new capacity to carry out this destruction.

A related phenomenon was discovered by a number of investigators about the same time in "agglutination," that is, the clumping and adhesion of bacteria or cells under the action of the serum of an animal immunized against them. In 1896 Max von Gruber and Herbert Durham found that bacteria isolated from a patient could be identified by their behavior with antiserum of known preparation. Fernand Widal reversed the procedure, noting that a patient's serum could be tested with bacteria of known type and his disease identified in this way. The well known Gruber-Widal test for typhoid fever was the outcome of these researches.

A closely related reaction was discovered in the following year by Rudolf Kraus, who found that when he mixed clear filtrates from bacterial cultures with antisera to the same bacteria, a cloudiness or precipitate occurred. He named this phenomenon the "precipitin reaction." Its sharp specificity soon made it useful in the identification of proteins, and particularly of blood stains.

All these discoveries threw a fresh light on the fluid elements of the body, and proved incontestably their great importance in disease. Thus the return to Hippocrates seemed complete. The proper concentration not of bile and mucus, to be sure, but of specific defensive substances in the humors of the body, prevented the development of contagious disease. However, the rival theory of solidism was already well under way. Élie Metchnikoff (1845-1916), a Russian at Odessa, had shown that amoeboid cells in fluids could engulf solid particles (1884). Attracted to the Pasteur Institute in Paris by the fame of Pasteur, Metchnikoff there soon showed that the leucocytes of the blood could and on occasion did engulf and destroy disease-producing bacteria. He gave his name "phagocytes" from κύτος, cell and φαγεῖν, to eat) to the cells, and "phagocytosis" to the process of bacterial engulfment. Thus arose the concept of body scavengers now familiar even to the schoolchild.

And so within the short space of a decade the mechanism of resistance to bacterial infection was twice explained and the issue confused. Buchner, Pfeiffer, and others had shown that blood could destroy bacteria to some extent before immunization had occurred, and still better afterwards. Metchnikoff proved the identical fact for his phagocytes. Both the so-called "native" or original immunity, and that acquired by specific immunization, could be explained on either ground. The solution of this seeming puzzle was promptly forthcoming, however, in the work of J. Denys and Leclef, who showed in 1895 that the serum of an animal immunized to a given disease in a remarkable fashion favored the activity of phagocytes toward the germ of that disease.

This work was confirmed by others, particularly Sir Almroth Wright and his associates, who proposed the term "opsonin" (from a Greek word meaning "I prepare") for the substance in the serum acting on the bacteria and rendering them susceptible to phagocytosis.

In this way the humoral and cellular doctrines of defense were largely reconciled. It remained for Paul Ehrlich (1854-1915) to bring the diverse phenomena of the two types of immunity into a single great working system. This was his famous "side-chain" theory, based on an analogy to the chemical side-chains of the aromatic hydrocarbons. Ehrlich likened the injured cells to these chemical compounds, endowed them with the capacity to take on and give up side-chains which had a protective capacity in the face of bacterial invasion, and thus established the now well-grounded concept of "antibodies" to disease germs and their poisons. An important feature of the theory, the sloughing of protective side chains in excess of the requirements of the immediate injury, was based on the fact of excessive tissue reparation following injury, to which attention had been called by Ehrlich's cousin Carl Weigert. Ehrlich's hypotheses have been much modified and certain specific concepts all but abandoned. But the stimulus given to immunology through his careful organization of its manifold phenomena has been of immeasurable value.

The new science of immunology was greatly advanced through the recognition of a number of special types of antibody manifestation. Jules Bordet, who developed a widely followed physico-chemical hypothesis of the immunity reactions in general, with Octave Gengou in 1900-2 made an important specific contribution in discovering that the serum of animals immunized to special red blood cells acquired the capacity to dissolve other cells of the same type. Their recognition of the rôle of two elements in this reaction, both contained in serum, viz., "antibody" and "serum complement," led to their development of the "complement-fixation reaction." A modification of this reaction, devised by August von Wassermann (1866-1925) in 1906, has had huge application in the diagnosis of syphilis.

It is now known that immunized animals whose serum gives evidence of the capacity to react in the complement-fixation and precipitin tests with the protein of the immunization, may be thrown into profound shock by injection of a small amount of that protein into the blood stream. The name "anaphylaxis" (from ἀνά and φυλάσσειν, guard against) was given to this phenomenon by Charles Richet in 1912. A series of related phenomena are today grouped under the broad terms "allergy" and "hypersensitiveness."

As readily seen, even from this brief summary of its most conspicuous phenomena, immunology in the first decades of its existence as a separate science had already reached an extraordinary degree of complexity, and its ramifications were being extended every hour.

While the development of bacteriology and immunology just described was taking place, equally productive investigations were being made in the related fields of human infection by non-bacterial parasites and the transmission of parasitic diseases. The parasite of malaria, one of the great scourges of the human race long recognized as a specific disease, was discovered in 1880 by Alphonse Laveran, a French army surgeon in Algiers. The manner of transmission remained clouded until 1897-98, when Ronald Ross in India discovered the part played by mosquitoes. The work was confirmed and extended by Giovanni Battista Grassi and other Italians, who demonstrated the rôle of the anopheles species of mosquito in human transmission.

A number of extremely important researches led up to these final achievements. Two discoveries had pointed the way for a recognition of insect transmission. In England, as early as 1879, Sir Patrick Manson had shown that the mosquito was the carrier of the parasite of the most common form of the tropical disease *filariasis*, and it was largely Manson's suggestions and encouragement that led to Ross's final success in malaria. Another pioneer discovery was the finding by Theobald Smith in America of the parasite of "Texas fever" in cattle and the recognition of its transfer from infected to well cattle by a cattle tick (1893).

The establishment of mosquito transmission as a fact in malaria opened the way for the solution of other tropical riddles. One of the most brilliant successes attended the efforts of an American army commission in 1900, composed of Walter Reed, James Carroll, Aristides Agramonte and Jesse W. Lazear, who traced the transmission of the unknown virus of yellow fever to mosquitoes of the species now known as *Aedes aegypti*. In the course of the rigorous and heroic tests to prove the theory Carroll acquired the disease in mild form and Lazear lost his life. In more recent years the insect transmission of numerous other diseases has been recognized, and through this recognition an effective means of control has been realized.

CHAPTER XII

Experimental and Chemical Pathology

The events recorded in the last chapter obviously opened up a new method of studying disease. Many abnormal states previously confined to man or occurring but sporadically in animals and of hitherto unknown cause could now be transmitted at will to laboratory animals and studied throughout their course. Thus bacteriology led directly into experimental pathology.

It must not be supposed, however, that the latter science was a new development. From the earliest times there has been an experimental pathology. The philosophers of antiquity realized as well as the physiologists of today the limitations of simple observation of life in its spontaneous course, and the necessity of controlled experiment for understanding certain facts.

Moreover, in antiquity superstition and religious prejudice went far to prevent that unrestricted observation of man and his inner ailments permitted by the free inquiry of a later day. For well over a thousand years the physiological and pathological concepts of the civilized world were based on the views of a man who gained most of his information through animal dissection and experiment, Galen, who saw the interior of only a few dead human bodies in his life.

It is true that Galen's experiments were devised for the elucidation of physiological problems but, as we shall see, no sharp line can be drawn between experiments designed to explain normal and disturbed function. In experimental science physiology and pathology become inseparable. This will be apparent when we note how Harvey's experimental demonstration of the circulation of the blood led directly to the explanation of one type of edema.

156

If experimental pathology was the only recourse of Galen, whose access to diseased human tissue was so restricted, it has proved no less expedient for those whose opportunities in this connection have been unlimited. Rokitansky, with seventy thousand necropsy protocols in his files, insisted that "Pathological anatomy, applying its methods of observation and investigation to the living body, requires an experimental pathology to establish the conditions surrounding the origin, existence, and involution of the anatomical disturbances it discovers." The enormous development of institutions specifically devoted to experimental pathology in the decades following this pronouncement, has amply borne him out.

Again, experiment has often proved the short cut to a knowledge far more slowly and haltingly acquired through chance observation. The immediate application of Harvey's methods to pathological problems, after his discovery of the circulation, illustrates this in an unmistakable way. The relation of a failing circulation to a swelling of the skin of the ankles and the development of general dropsy must have been vaguely realized after it was demonstrated that the blood did circulate, and even before that (see Pieter Pauw's observation, page 53). But it remained for Richard Lower (1631-1691) of London to prove the relationship, which he did by very simple experimentation.

Lower's many animal experiments, described in his *Tractatus de corde* (1669, forty-one years after the first appearance of Harvey's epoch-making work), include many devoted to the results of stagnation of the venous circulation, produced by compression or iigature of veins. Instead of finding extravasated blood, as he expected, on opening the greatly swollen parts distal to the pressure, he found the tissues filled with serum, in short, of that appearance often observed in human dropsy. Cautiously, he refused to make the application until he had ligated the vena cava above the diaphragm in a dog and seen the development of ascites. This experiment, of two days' duration, was indeed a short cut to a major piece of information.

Nor was such useful animal experimentation by any means confined to circulatory disturbances. A contemporary of Lower, Johann Conrad Brunner (1653-1727), discoverer of the duodenal glands that bear his name, was much occupied with the function of the abdominal viscera, particularly those related to the digestive tract. In a number of dogs he removed the pancreas, a piece of good operating for its day, and was much interested in the fact that after the operation these dogs were hungrier than before, were excessively thirsty and voided urine frequently. His experiment was too far ahead of the times for perfect understanding, however. Had the methods of chemical analysis of the nineteenth century been available he would have been the first to discover pancreatic diabetes. His dogs were certainly in the diabetic state.

These are but two of many who were using the experimental method for gaining desired biological information. It is only because of the isolated individuality of such efforts that any justification is found for the special emphasis laid upon the pioneer experimental investigations of a later period. Rival nations have united in assigning the foundership of modern experimental pathology to John Hunter. If this position is truly merited, it is on the ground of his incessant insistence on resort to experiment when other means failed. He carried out every sort of experiment himself, and, other animals failing, used his own person. He broke his health with long hours of experimental labor. Yet he introduced no new method of approach to pathology; he simply made the value of the experimental method so certain by indefatigable persistence in its application that it could never again lose its place.

Virchow, who credited Hunter with this establishment of experimental pathology, made extensive use of its practice himself. In his great work on embolism he constantly supported his deductions from his post-mortem anatomical discoveries by attempts to reproduce the lesions experimentally. This effort struck the very keynote of modern experimental pathology. The accurate and regular artificial reproduction of a lesion hitherto obscure is often sought as the surest way of learning its natural cause. Virchow's intravascular injections of pieces of real thrombi and of tissue and of air and fat and even fine particles of starch, probably had as much to do with his final understanding of the occurrence and manifestations of embolism as his dissection of dead bodies.

His colleague Ludwig Traube (1818-1876), trained in Breslau by Purkinje and in Berlin by Johannes Müller and Schönlein, had already launched a journal which was to be devoted more or less exclusively to the results of experimental methods in pathology, the *Beiträge zur experimentellen Pathologie*. Traube had originally planned to devote his attention to the usual types of clinical observation, but an administrative order in the hospital cutting off his supply of patients for study, he turned his energy to animal experimentation. His most important achievement was the recognition of the pulmonary disorders occurring after cutting the vagus nerves. Although his *Beiträge* was of short life, his influence remained profound, and after the revolution of 1848 had restored his clinical opportunities, his professional rise was rapid. He became a very popular teacher of clinical medicine, his precise information resting largely on his experiments.

The early investigations of Recklinghausen have already been mentioned. This able pupil of Virchow was one of his teacher's staunchest supporters with regard to the pus cell, which Virchow considered a local tissue cell. Although Recklinghausen's own moist chamber experiments of 1863 on the amoeboid motility of the leucocytes had strongly indicated the relationship of the white blood corpuscle to the pus cell, his experiments of 1867 on inflammation of the frog cornea seemed to prove that pus and its specific cells could arise from preëxisting tissue cells. And strange as it may seem, it was on the lowly frog's cornea that the great, age-long battle over the nature of inflammation was finally fought to a finish.

In the same year as Recklinghausen's publication, Vol. 40 of Virchow's *Archiv* opened with the revolutionary article of Julius Cohnheim entitled *Ueber Entzündung und Eiterung*. Cohnheim (1839-1884), perhaps the most distinguished of the many celebrated pupils of Virchow, a Pomeranian by birth like his teacher, was assistant to the latter in Berlin from 1864-68. Like many of the well trained German pathologists, he had devoted his first interest to normal histology and neurology, developing a beautiful technic, afterwards to serve him in good stead. His attention was soon caught by pathological problems, in the course of which he devised a number of happy experiments for studying inflammation.

Following Recklinghausen's lead he first worked on the cornea of the frog. In their completed form the steps of the experiment were as follows. He stained the aqueous humor of the anterior chamber with aniline blue. Incoming leucocytes acquired the blue color. Then he irritated the cornea. Soon new cells resembling leucocytes made their appearance in the injured cornea. They were not blue, but white. Therefore, they had not come from the neighboring anterior chamber. Next he injected dyes into the frog's dorsal lymph sac, a procedure resulting in the staining of a large number of white corpuscles which ultimately found their way into the blood stream. He again injured the cornea and this time stained corpuscles appeared at the site of irritation.

The proof seemed complete that the pus corpuscles in a zone of injury came from the blood, but Cohnheim wished to make doubly sure. He desired to see the corpuscles in transit. To accomplish this he hit upon the expedient of using the delicate and transparent mesentery of the frog. The experiment is now a common one. Spreading this out on a warm, moist slide, or a ring of cork, so that the thin vessels could be watched under a microscope, he applied the irritating substance cantharidin to a portion of the tissue, after which he observed a marvelous change. The vessels widened, the current slowed, the red and white corpuscles, previously indistinguishable in the swift stream, became readily visible, and presently he observed the. astonishing fact of actual passage of blood leucocytes through the capillary walls and accumulation at the site of the injury. The conclusion was inescapable. The pus cells, that is the white cells found in regions of inflammation, were blood leucocytes. The blood vessels on which the ancients had laid such stress in inflammation were back in the foreground after Virchow's relegation in favor of the essentiality of local cellular change. *"Ohne Gefässe keine Entzündung,"* concluded Cohnheim.

The struggle was by no means over, however. A new champion for the old view appeared, Salomon Stricker (1834-1898) of Vienna, Hungarian-born, for whom a special chair of experimental pathology had been created on recognition of his talent by Rokitansky. Stricker's expert histological technic, which had resulted in his discovery in 1865 of diapedesis of the red blood cells through the capillaries, especially qualified him to meet Cohnheim on his own ground. Back to the cornea he went. He irritated it with lunar caustic and, examining the injured area quickly, found the local cells undergoing an almost immediate change, putting out processes and multiplying before any cells from the capillaries around the avascular cornea could possibly reach the site. The accumulation of these cells virtually constituted a region of pus.

Many others took a hand in the argument, which lasted for some years. Metchnikoff's distinction of small and large phagocytes did much to clear the air. Cohnheim's view that the leucocytes were pushed through the capillary walls was modified in favor of the modern notion of chemotaxis, or chemical attraction. Finally enough credit was left for all, in the recognition that in inflammatory processes local tissue cells, to which a

PLATE XLV

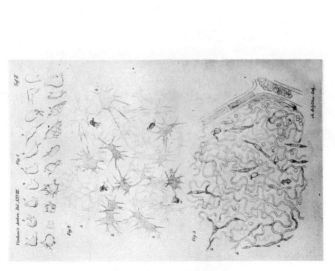

AMOEBOID CELLS
From Recklinghausen's *Ueber Eiter- und*
Bindegewebskörperchen, 1863

PLATE XLVI

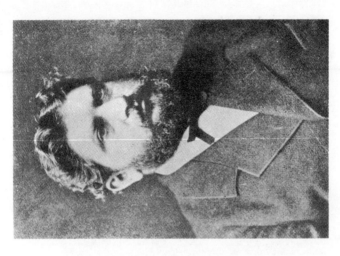

JULIUS COHNHEIM (1839-1884)

PLATE XLVII

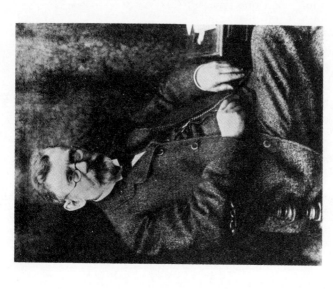

PAUL EHRLICH (1854-1915)
Courtesy of National Library of Medicine

PLATE XLVII

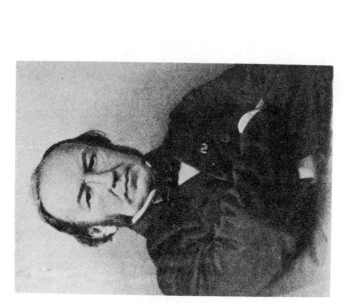

CLAUDE BERNARD (1813-1878)

variety of names have been given, and incoming colorless corpuscles of more than one type, all take part.

Cohnheim left his mark in many fields, chiefly by experimental methods. His successful inoculation of tuberculosis in the anterior chamber of a rabbit's eye, where the process of development of the disease could be observed through the transparent cornea, convinced the doubting scientific world of the infectiousness of the disease and left the isolation of its causative virus only a question of time.

In 1872 appeared his epoch-making *Investigations on the Embolic Processes.* In this he developed the doctrine of infarction as a result of occlusion of terminal arteries ("*Endarterien*"), explaining the hemorrhagic nature of certain infarcts on the basis of a reflux flow from the veins and diapedesis through the altered capillaries of the infarcted area. Previously the phenomenon of infarction had been attributed to capillary occlusion in the region involved.

Through these masterly achievements Cohnheim became the leader in experimental pathology in Europe, and second only to Virchow in his influence upon general pathology. Among the many students who sought his laboratory was William Welch, whose own later extended consideration of the subjects of thrombosis, embolism, and infarction and important articles on venous thrombosis in cardiac disease did much to further the understanding of these circulatory derangements. Welch was in Breslau in its most brilliant period. Cohnheim was occupied with his tumor theory and the compilation of his *Lectures on General Pathology,* Weigert was making most of the necropsies, Ehrlich as a young student was already, almost literally, deep in aniline dyes. Cohn and Heidenhain were attracting eager students in botany, bacteriology, and physiology. Koch had made his great anthrax demonstration there but a few months before. At Cohnheim's suggestion Welch undertook an investigation on acute edema of the lungs, which led him to conclude that this familiar condition could result from a disproportion in the working power of the two ventricles of the heart.

Back in America after a tour that brought him into contact with Klebs, Stricker, Heschl, Chiari, Rindfleisch, Ziegler, and Recklinghausen, Welch definitely entered the field of pathology and soon occupied the chair in the subject at Johns Hopkins University. It was now the period of most intense development in bacteriology, and in this field, too, Welch took his place among the pioneers through his discovery with Nuttall, of the gas bacillus (*Bacillus aerogenes capsulatus,* Welch's bacillus). In the succeeding years he remained a guiding force in medical education and research in the United States.

In France the experimental method was yielding results of the first importance in a quite different field. The outstanding figure was Claude Bernard (1813-1878), who had come to Paris as a hopeful dramatist and remained to become the master physiologist of his time. Kindly advice and a shift to medicine, where he came under the influence of the physiologist Magendie, initiated the change. But where Magendie was content with physiology for its own sake, Bernard was more largely concerned with its application to disease. His point of view is well illustrated in his stimulating book *Experimental Medicine,* written in the leisure hours of convalescence from a serious illness.

Bernard's discovery of the part played by the liver in regulating sugar metabolism through its function of storing glycogen (1843-57) was the foundation of our knowledge of the "organs of internal secretion," and has proved of great importance in our present conceptions of diabetes mellitus. His work on the pancreatic juice (1849-56) opened up a new understanding of the physiology, and secondarily of the pathology of digestion. His third discovery, the vasomotor mechanism, so important for normal physiology, finds many applications in pathology, in the understanding of the condition of active hyperemia, perhaps of angina pectoris, and many states where the line between pathology and physiology cannot be sharply drawn.

His successor in experimental medicine in Paris, Charles-Édouard Brown-Séquard (1817-1894), a native of Mauritius, of American-French parentage, who spent much of his life in the United States, still further developed the field of internal secretions. Shortly after Addison's discovery of the serious constitutional disease associated with lesions of the suprarenal glands, he confirmed Addison's conclusion of their importance for the maintenance of life, by the production of severe symptoms and rapid death through their removal in animals. His belief in the effects of internal secretion led him to attempt the alleviation of the manifestations of advancing age by the injection of organ extracts, and more rationally to try the same method in acromegaly, which his countryman Marie and others had traced to abnormality of another ductless gland, the hypophysis. Brown-Séquard had already followed the trend of French pathology by taking up neuropathology, using the experimental method. His hemisections and transections of the spinal cord helped in an understanding of the symptoms of some of the naturally arising lesions of this organ, and left his name attached to one particular nervous syndrome, hemiplegia with anesthesia of the opposite side.

The conception of internal secretion goes back to the time of Théophile de Bordeu (1722-1776), a celebrated Paris physician, who maintained that each organ elaborated a specific product which passed into the blood stream. Today the concept is usually limited to those glands without an external secretion, which are known to play an important part in animal metabolism, particularly the thyroid, parathyroids, hypophysis, pancreas in part, adrenals, and the sex glands. The simple theory of Bordeu has been carried on to an extraordinary degree of refinement; today the internal secretion of most of the glands has been isolated, and a remarkable correlation between certain internally secreting glands established.

Observations on abnormalities of these glands and associated metabolic disorder are more than a century old. The best known instance is that of exophthalmic goiter, eight cases of which were studied by Caleb Parry of Bath (1755-1822) between 1786 and 1815. It was later described in detail by Robert James Graves (1835) and by Karl von Basedow in Germany (1840).

Much of our present knowledge of the function of the ductless glands has been derived from a study of the results of their extirpation in animals. The zoölogist and physiologist Moritz Schiff (1823-1896) recorded the development of that series of symptoms we now recognize as associated with thyroid insufficiency, following experimental excision of the gland in dogs (1856 ff.). In 1883 the surgeon Theodor Kocher of Bern (1841-1917) reported unintentional experiments of the same character in man, describing the metabolic disorders occurring in a number of his own patients following the surgical removal of the thyroid for other disease. Sir William Gull in England described the symptom complex of thyroid insufficiency from other causes in man in 1873.

In the same volume of the journal in which Basedow's classic account of hyperthyroidism appeared (1840), an observation was published by Bernhard Mohr of that remarkable type of obesity now known as "Fröhlich's syndrome" (from the description by Alfred Fröhlich in 1901). At autopsy a degenerating tumor of the hypophysis was found. We have already noted the relation of this organ to gigantism and the condition of acromegaly. We have also noted Addison's discovery of the fatal issue of chronic disease of the anatomically inconspicuous adrenal glands. The elucidation of the part played by the pancreas in normal metabolism, one of the triumphs of modern physiology, largely explained the nature of diabetes.

Physiological dysfunction in its relation to specific organ pathology was studied with great vigor by a group of German clinicians during the second half of the nineteenth century. The chief guide and mentor was Friedrich Theodor von Frerichs (1819-1885), a Göttingen graduate whose fruitful labors and effective teaching in the medical clinics of Kiel and Breslau led to his call to Berlin in 1859 to succeed Schönlein, who had been one of the most influential teachers Germany ever possessed. Frerichs' important studies included notable inquiries into Bright's disease, uremic intoxication, diabetes, and malaria. He is particularly remembered, however, for his extensive investigations on diseases of the liver. He published two quite distinct monographs under the title *Klinik der Leberkrankheiten,* which summarized the history and existing knowledge with respect to this organ and added Frerichs' own brilliant contributions. The degenerative condition known as acute yellow atrophy was treated at length, Frerichs calling attention to the excretion of excessive quantities of leucine and tyrosine and their presence in the urine in crystalline form as pathognomonic for the disease.

His most important experimental investigations were on jaundice, in which he ligated the ductus choledochus, injected the bile constituents, etc., drawing conclusions which, however, have not been entirely substantiated. He was much interested in the fatty liver, and demonstrated a partial relationship between the diet and its origin. He used the best chemical methods constantly, and may be considered as much an early leader of chemical pathology as of experimental. His analyses of gallstones stimulated his pupil Bernard Naunyn (1839-1925) to develop the chemical aspects of this field and devise an accurate chemical classification.

The keen rivalry over patients for study in the Charité Hospital brought him the lasting dislike of Virchow and Traube, which was not shared, however, by the students, of whom von Mering, Ehrlich, and Naunyn may be reckoned as his greatest, Naunyn following out most closely the lines he had laid down.

One of the most brilliant achievements of the Frerichs school was the artificial production of pancreatic diabetes by Josef von Mering (1849-1907) and Oscar Minkowski, who recognized the manifestations of diabetes after excision of the pancreas in dogs, and cleared the way for the equally notable advances of modern medicine in the study and treatment of this disease.

The leading exponent of chemical and experimental pathology and their related fields in recent times has without doubt been Paul Ehrlich (1854-1915), assistant of Frerichs from 1878-85, whose services to immunology have already been mentioned. Trained originally in the Breslau school, where Weigert's technic in differential staining much impressed him, he made out of staining and the theory of dyes, which had seemed little more than a hobby to his Breslau associates, a foundation broad enough to support several new and major sciences, including hematology, immunology, and chemotherapy. His separation of the different kinds of leucocytes according to their individual staining capacity, and his discovery of the acid-fastness of the tubercle bacillus, in the same year that Koch discovered the germ, were masterly achievements in the field of microchemical analysis. His studies on the blood laid the foundations for our present differentiations in the fields of anemia and leukemia.

He was a fertile chemist with a capacity for bold generalization. He took over the Kekulé theory for the structure of benzene, about which much of the science of organic chemistry had been built, and constructed around it a comprehensive theory for the new, and largely his own, science of immunology.

Dyes again furnished the medium for his development of chemotherapy. His intravital selective staining of cells and their invaders led him to the ambitious project of making modified dyes, containing a germicidal chemical group, with the same selective affinity for the germs within the tissues. His attack on the spirochete of syphilis according to this principle, in which one fortified dye after another was tried and discarded, until over six hundred lay on the scrap heap, but a six hundred and sixth proved potent, is one of the great and inspiring stories of medicine.

The increasing assistance of chemistry to pathology makes it desirable at this point to go back and trace some of the development of its biological branch which, like physiology, can never be considered wholly separate from pathology. We have seen that as far back as the alchemistic age van Helmont developed the fruitful theory of special ferments. Many of the great pathological anatomists used the methods of chemical analysis, generally beginning with that keen method which has since been discarded for others less likely to give offense, the sense of taste. Morgagni boiled specimens of the effusions he encountered in the serous cavities, noting with care the character of the coagulum, Bright inaugurated a new epoch through his combination of pathological anatomy and urinary analysis. Andral and others pioneered in the applications of blood chemistry to pathology, Rokitansky avowed chemical pathology to be the pathology of the future, and Virchow, the cellular pathologist, corrected Rokitansky's chemical errors.

Organized chemical pathology depended on more concerted effort, however. And this began with the great development of chemical laboratories in Germany in the second quarter of the nineteenth century, under the influence of Justus von Liebig (1803-1873), a pupil of the French chemical school of Gay-Lussac. From this fruitful period organic chemistry took its start. Moreover, the barriers between this kind of chemistry and the chemistry of the living body were broken down almost as soon as they were set up, by Friedrich Wöhler's (1800-1882) laboratory conversion (1828) of the organic substance ammonium cyanate into urea, a typical animal substance, the chief end product of nitrogen metabolism in the human body. Other discoveries of the utmost physiological importance followed in rapid succession in the hands of Liebig, Wöhler, and their associates and pupils.

A huge development of chemical physiology and pathology was fostered by Felix Hoppe-Seyler (1825-1895), whose early training was medical, and who for eight years was an assistant of Virchow in the Pathological Institute of Berlin. Hoppe-Seyler founded the profoundly influential *Zeitschrift für physiologische Chemie* (1877) and wrote the textbook of physiological chemistry (1877-81) on which the first generation of investigators in this field were brought up.

The leading physiological chemist of later times, and one of the greatest chemists of all time, was Emil Fischer (1852-1919), for a quarter of a century professor in Berlin, who advanced every field of biological chemistry by direct personal investigation as well as through the training of a host of brilliant pupils. The carbohydrate and protein chemistry of today is largely Fischer chemistry. His elucidation of the structure of the proteins, his methods of protein analysis, and finally his resynthesis of the protein "building blocks" into molecularly huge, protein-like compounds, were spectacular, and have proved of far-reaching consequence, as it is the proteins, of all chemical compounds, that appear peculiarly characteristic of life and living processes.

The new approach to physiological and pathological understanding made possible through this chemical development brought fresh and vigorous reinforcement into fields where advance through morphological research seemingly approached an end.

The problem of edema, as old and sore a one as inflammation, over which the pathological anatomists and physiologists of centuries have stumbled, received new light from the investigations of modern physical chemistry on osmotic pressure and the hydration of colloids. Without chemistry there would be little understanding of necrosis, suppuration, gangrene and the degenerative lesions in general, subjects to which the slowly acquired knowledge of tissue ferments has brought much explanation. The many and varied processes involved in calcification of lesions and in concretion formation, once somewhat facetiously isolated as geological, or more appropriately mineralogical pathology, are obviously in the field of the chemical branch.

The immunologists have looked to the colloid chemists to solve their most pressing problems. A new science arose in the recognition of a lack of certain growth-promoting substances, or vitamins, as the basis of a set of diseases of a nature hitherto unknown. Probably in no field, however, has more substantial aid been brought than in that of the intoxications. The hopeful beginnings of Bright, Bostock, and Andral have been succeeded by a science of blood chemistry of monumental proportions with corresponding increase in the understanding of uremia, diabetes, and a variety of forms of acidosis. Easy chemical methods of following the course of metabolism in the human body now detect and make understandable disturbances in function quite beyond the range of the older pathology.

It is not inappropriate to close this book with this brief recital of the achievements of chemistry, for on this science unquestionably depends much of the advance of pathology in the future. We have seen how the subject of pathology was taken out of the realm of speculation by the rational investigation of the pathological anatomists of the sixteenth, seventeenth, and eighteenth centuries. We have seen that organ pathology became tissue pathology, and tissue pathology again cellular pathology, thanks to the rise of cytology and histology. The science of bacteriology brought new methods and new points of view. It is inevitable that refinements of our growing natural science will find further application in our pathology of the future, as they always have in the past. It is but natural to suppose that the attention which has successively, and with profit, been focussed on diseased organs, diseased tissues, and diseased cells, can with considerable prospect of success be concentrated on the still mysterious colloidal emulsion within the cell itself. The increasing facilities granted for the advance of chemical methods in the great institutes of medical research testify to a rather general recognition of this view.

Yet there is no present warrant for predicting any change so revolutionary as the cellular doctrine of the nineteenth century. Although it is difficult if not impossible to evaluate the progress of our own generation, there is much to indicate that the modern spirit of pathology is expressed in organization and that present advance is being brought about as much through well-designed administration as that individual capacity which proved so fertile in the preceding century. The rapid extension of the literature of the science, the constant revision of many able texts, the sharp demarcation of fields by excellent reviews and monographs, have all combined to make the uncertainties and deficiences in our knowledge conspicuous.

The World War of 1914-1918, which showed the vital importance of executive detail in scientific research as well as military operations, had its aftermath in improved organization of all scientific investigation. Leaders in pathology, as well as other sciences, through their students launched well-developed attacks deliberately calculated to fill the gaps in existing knowledge. The well-known, highly effective organization of Ludwig Aschoff in Germany for teaching and research may be cited as an example of this trend. Capable administration and the recognition of fruitful projects, although less dramatic, thus apparently become as important in the furtherance of knowledge in pathology as individual investigative originality.

Bibliography

The following works have been of exceptional influence on the development of pathology, and are recommended for further reading as a short set of classics in this subject:

The Works of HIPPOCRATES. (Fourth Century B.C.) (English translation by W. H. S. Jones and E. T. Withington (1923 ff).

CELSUS, CORNELIUS. *De Re Medicina.* (First Century A.D.) (English translation by James Greive, 1756.)

THE WORKS OF GALEN. (Second Century A.D.) (French translation by Ch. Daremberg, 1854-56).

BENIVIENI, ANTONIO. *De Abditis Nonnullis ac Mirandis Morborum et Sanationum Causis* (1507). (Translation by Singer in Singer, C., and Long, E.R., *Benivieni. The Hidden Causes of Disease,* C. C Thomas, Springfield, Ill., 1954.)

FERNEL, JEAN. *Medicina. Pathologiae Libri VII* (1554).

TULP, NICOLAES. *Observationum Medicarum Libri IV* (1641).

WEPFER, JOHANN JAKOB. *Observationes Anatomicae ex Cadaveribus Eorum Quos Sustulit Apoplexia* (1658).

SYLVIUS, FRANCISCUS (FRANZ DE LE BOË). *De Phthisi (Opera Medica,* 1679.)

BONET, THÉOPHILE. *Sepulchretum sive Anatomia Practica* (1679).

RUYSCH, FREDERIK. *Thesaurus Anatomicus* (1701-15). *Observationum Anatomico-Chirurgicarum Centuria* (1691-1737.)

MORGAGNI, GIOVANNI BATTISTA. *De Sedibus et Causis Morborum* (1761). (English translation by Benjamin Alexander, 1769; reprinted, with additions by P. Klemperer, Hafner Publishing Co., New York, 1960.)

HUNTER, JOHN. *Treatise on the Blood, Inflammation and Gunshot Wounds* (1794).

BAILLIE, MATTHEW. *The Morbid Anatomy of Some of the Most Important Parts of the Human Body* (1794).

BICHAT, XAVIER. *Anatomie Générale* (1801). (English translation by George Hayward, 1822.)

LAËNNEC, RENÉ-THÉOPHILE-HYACINTHE. *Traité de l'Auscultation Médiate* (1819). (English translation of selected passages by Sir William Hale-White, 1923.)

BRIGHT, RICHARD. *Reports of Medical Cases* (1827).

CRUVEILHIER, JEAN. *Anatomie Pathologique du Corps Humain ou Descriptions avec Figures Lithographiées et Coloriées des Diverses Altérations Morbides* (1829-42).

ROKITANSKY, CARL. *Lehrbuch der pathologischen Anatomie* (1842-46). (English translation by Sydenham Society, 1849-54).

ADDISON, THOMAS. *On the Constitutional and Local Effects of Disease of the Suprarenal Capsules* (1855).

VIRCHOW, RUDOLF. *Die Cellularpathologie in ihrer Begründung auf physiologische und pathologische Gewebelehre* (1858). (English translation by Frank Chance, 1863.)

COHNHEIM, JULIUS. *Ueber Eiterung und Entzündung* (Virchow's *Archiv*, 1867).

Two important and stimulating textbooks of pathological anatomy written in the United States in the early years of the nineteenth century, indicate the early advanced point of view in this country:

HORNER, WILLIAM EDMONDS. *A Treatise on Pathological Anatomy* (Philadelphia, 1829).

GROSS, SAMUEL D. *Elements of Pathological Anatomy* (Boston, 1839).

APPENDIX

Recent Trends in Pathology, 1929-1963

In 1958 pathological laboratories and institutes around the world celebrated the centennial of Rudolf Virchow's publication of *Die Cellularpathologie*. The profound influence of this work on the understanding and development of pathology was everywhere recognized, and many distinguished pathologists used the occasion for an appraisal of the state of pathology in their time in comparison with its stage of development before the advent of the cellular doctrine.

In a similar way, the original edition of *A History of Pathology* noted the significance of the revolution introduced by the cellular pathology, as seen after seventy years, and in Chapter IX the dominant rôle played by Virchow and his pupils in the latter years of the nineteenth century was emphasized. While gazing somewhat cautiously toward the future, the author saw no reason at that time for predicting in the foreseeable part of the twentieth century any change so revolutionary as the cellular doctrine of the middle of the nineteenth.

Yet even in the tribute paid by the writer of this book to Virchow's influence and the master rôle of cellular pathology in the science of pathology as a whole, the opinion was hazarded that after a long course of history during which organ pathology had become tissue pathology, and the latter, in turn, cellular pathology, it seemed but natural to suppose that the attention which had been focussed successively and with profit on diseased organs, diseased tissues, and diseased cells, might in time, with some prospect of success, be concentrated on the still mysterious colloidal emulsion within the cell itself (page 168).

As it actually turned out, a century after the cellular pathology had revolutionized the science, the development of a molecular pathology, supplementing, although by no means supplanting, the cellular concept of the science, was truly under way. The evolution was due in large measure to technical advances in other fields. Biochemistry, in its applications to normal physiology and disease processes as well, had made great strides in the interval, and technical improvements in the visual perception of structures concerned had undergone a parallel development. The electron microscope, the most conspicuous among numerous advances in the enlargement of fine structures for visual study, had made it possible to see changes that could only be imagined at the time the cellular doctrine was promulgated. This electronic device at the present writing is as yet far from being the indispensable instrument that light microscopes have been during the last century, but an inescapable similarity is evident in the papers presented in pathological societies today to the exciting, if still crude, pictures presented by Lebert, Vogel, Gerlach and other histologists at corresponding meetings a century and more ago.

Microscopic studies, in turn, it should be noted, have been supplemented by refined "ultra" chemical methods, including spectroscopy, electrophoretic and ultra-centrifuge procedures, and chromatography, for the identification and measurement of minute structures and significant components of body fluids.

In this evolution pathology as a medical discipline has lost a little of the status it enjoyed when the master pathological anatomists of bygone years were able to reserve for themselves an authoritarian and frequently finalizing attitude toward the older clinicians, whose diagnoses, without such modern aids as x-ray photography, electrocardiography and clinical laboratory procedures, more often then than now, were mistaken.

INTEGRATION OF PATHOLOGY
WITH OTHER SCIENCES

In the course of a quite natural process of amalgamation, pathology has now become integrated with other sciences and a more general discipline of microbiology. Indeed academic departments and institutions once designated as organizations for pathology and bacteriology, have now, in the light of advances in chemistry, immunology, and microscopy, and new knowledge of viral and parasitic disease, become correspondingly organizations of "pathology and microbiology."

Few developments today have exceeded in their productiveness the understanding that has been achieved of the nature of the minute, genetically vital nuclear and cytoplasmic compounds, desoxyribonucleic acid (DNA) and ribonucleic acid (RNA) and the part they play in the synthesis of cellular proteins. At the time of writing, it is conceived that proteins are synthesized from their small constituent building blocks in the surrounding plasma on frameworks of nucleic acid, supplied with enzymic mechanisms determining protein specificity through the order in which amino acids are incorporated—an informational procedure known as genetic coding. Among the protein complexes so synthesized, in current theory, are antibodies important in the body's resistance to disease. Where the new knowledge will lead is as yet impossible to predict, but current conception of its possibilities is reflected in the emphasis laid in a continuing stream of Nobel prizes in this field of physiology and medicine. As perhaps minor illustrations of possibilities for pathology, the chemical and visual recognition of a chromosomal basis for such diverse abnormalities as hemophilia, mongolism, and intersexual states may be mentioned.

Much of the new knowledge has come about through advances in histochemistry, a field of new emphasis, which takes advantage of such procedures as differential staining for enzyme activity, vital staining, fluorescence microscopy and autoradiography following the use of radioactive isotopes. The isotopes, following the pioneer studies of Georg von Hevesy of Budapest, at Niels Bohr's Institute for Theoretical Physics in Copenhagen (1923 ff.), have proved of inestimable value as biological tracers in studying metabolism and metabolic disorders. It is believed that in such extensions of intimacy in the examination of diseased body parts, a closer approximation to the phenomena of disordered function has been achieved than was ever before possible.

Of somewhat comparable interest are technics for artificial culture of tissues that have been developed during the twentieth century. These stem back to early successes in tissue culture by R. G. Harrison in New Haven with nerve cells (1907 ff.) and Alexis Carrel in New York with tumor cells and connective and other tissues (1910 ff.). These accomplishments, in later years, paved the way for studies of tumor growth, immunology, and other aspects of pathology.

In general, the advances in pathology that have taken place in the period since that outlined in the last chapter of *A History of Pathology* have been in those fields that gave that chapter its title, viz., experimental and chemical pathology. Briefly, and without much attempt to pinpoint discoveries on which subsequent progress was based, and no attempt to be comprehensive in any field, an effort will now be made to indicate, by example, subjects in which conspicuous advances have been made—taking them up more or less in the time-honored way followed in text-books of pathology, and beginning, perhaps appropriately, with the phenomena of inflammation.

INFLAMMATION

Attention may well be called here to the understanding brought about among medical students of the current century by a great teacher, J. G. Adami in Montreal, whose review mono-graph on the subject was widely read in the opening years of this century. Among concepts of particular interest that have developed since then is that of the reticulo-endothelial system, set forth by Ludwig Aschoff of Freiburg and his associates in 1913 and succeeding years, in which the rôles played by fixed tissue phagocytes throughout the body were abundantly demon-strated. Some explanation of the several bizarre lipoidoses, it may be noted, came about through an understanding of the reticulo-endothelial system.

Another concept, in the development of which many investi-gators have taken part, is that of allergic inflammation, in which an inflammatory reaction is envisioned as triggered by the meet-ing of antigenic substances and sensitized tissues at individual sites or more generally throughout the body. Intimately con-nected with the phenomena of inflammation are those of sus-ceptibility, resistance, and immunity. Included among the factors concerned are the humoral antibodies stimulated by disease or antigenic inoculation. A long search for the site of antibody production, much of it mediated by the fluorescent antibody technic of Coons of Boston, has taken place. At the time of writing, attention is focussed on a particular stage of develop-ment of the plasma cell.

INFECTIOUS AND PARASITIC DISEASE

A major field in which progress has been made is that of in-fectious and parasitic disease. Throughout the first half of the twentieth century, knowledge accumulated on the rôle of pyo-genic cocci in disease, including demonstration of an etiological relation between hemolytic streptococci and scarlet fever, of a

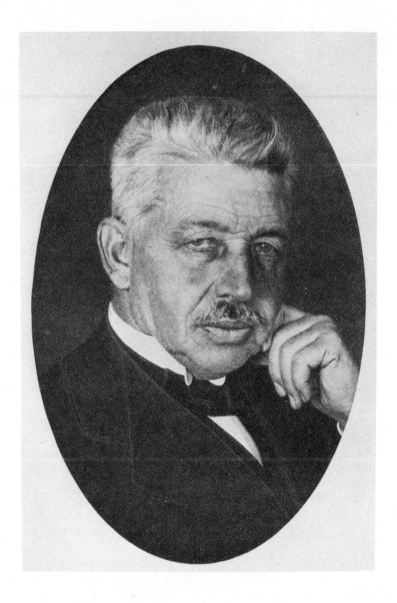

LUDWIG ASCHOFF (1866-1942)
Courtesy of National Library of Medicine

variety of types of pneumococci in pneumonia and of the variable pathogenicity of staphylococci, which display enhanced virulence at times in epidemics and cross infections in hospitals. In World War I (1914-18) the deadly rôle of anaerobic infection of wounds was conspicuous. Yet during all these years a rather general decrease in the prevalence and severity of certain bacterial diseases occurred, partly as a consequence of new methods in therapy and public health. Noteworthy declines have occurred in the relative frequency with which pathologists in their daily experience encounter cases of typhoid fever, lobar pneumonia, pulmonary tuberculosis, destructive syphilis, and bacterial endocarditis.

During the middle years of the first half of the century, important contributions were made on a variety of less well-known bacterial and virus diseases, including tularemia, brucellosis, and the ornithoses. Many of these were made in the Hygienic Laboratory of the U. S. Public Health Service.

One of the most remarkable developments during this period was the establishment of the etiology of what are now known as the rickettsial diseases. Early work in this field was in large part the outgrowth of American studies, in which the pioneer investigations of H. T. Ricketts on Rocky Mountain spotted fever and Mexican typhus fever (1910) were preëminent. Typhus fever was a scourge in some of the armies of World War I, and a related rickettsial disease, scrub typhus, or tsutsugamushi disease, had a similar military significance in World War II.

The preceding section of this book drew attention to the last third of the nineteenth century as the period of rapid development of bacteriology. The middle third of the twentieth century proved to be a corresponding period in understanding the relation of filterable viruses to disease. During this period major emphasis in the study of acute infectious disease, as reported in contemporary journals, has been on viruses rather than bacteria. The development of methods of cultivating viruses on living cells, in which E. W. Goodpasture in Nashville and his associates (1931 ff.) pioneered, was especially important. In succeeding years the viruses of many specific diseases, including poliomyelitis, influenza and yellow fever, were cultivated. The history of influenza is dramatic in this respect. The pandemic of 1918 stimulated extensive research. The discovery of its viral etiology by W. Smith, C. H. Andrews, and P. P. Laidlaw in England in experiments with ferrets (1933), and the later accomplishment of its artificial cultivation in the chick embryo, paved the way for many subsequent investigations. During World War II (1939-45) another viral disease, so-called atypical pneumonia, a much milder ailment, was pandemic. Other respiratory viruses became the subject of intensive investigations. "Infectious" hepatitis was a somewhat similar scourge in military experience and in more general epidemics; two varieties were prominent, epidemic hepatitis, spread by natural channels, and a dangerous type commonly transmitted by transfusions of what proved to be infected blood.

In this connection, note should be made of pioneer studies on the exact nature of a plant virus, that of tobacco mosaic disease. W. M. Stanley of the Rockefeller Institute in Princeton identified this in electron microscope studies (1935) and later crystallized it by chemical procedures. This advance paved the way for progress in the delineation of other viruses. Coupled with study of viruses has been the accumulation of much information on the vectors transmitting them.

Throughout all this period steady progress was made in knowledge of mycotic and animal parasitic disease. Elucidation of these world-wide diseases was gained from many sources. Typical examples were the study of coccidioidomycosis by investigators in regions of California where the disease was endemic, and that of histoplasmosis, first recognized, although imperfectly, by S. T. Darling in the Canal Zone of Panama (1902).

NUTRITIONAL AND TOXIC DISEASES

Spectacular advance has been made in the twentieth century in the understanding of nutritional diseases. Much of the progress was due to recognition of the role of vitamins in maintaining a normal nutritional state. Early studies included those on beri-beri by Christiaan Eijkman in Java (1890 ff.) and the Polish chemist Casimir Funk (1911 ff.), who proposed the name "vitamine." The field was widely cultivated by F. Gowland Hopkins at Cambridge (1906 ff.), who noted that animals could not live on protein, fat and carbohydrate alone, but needed, in addition, what he termed "accessory substances." American investigators, including E. V. McCollum in Madison and Baltimore, T. B. Osborne and L. B. Mendel in New Haven and S. B. Wolbach in Boston, developed a broad understanding of vitamin A and other deficiencies. The essential rôle of a dietary factor in rickets was recognized in England in 1918 by E. Mellanby. These are but a few of the many investigators whose work has been of historical significance in this large field.

Industrial hazards to health have occupied much of the attention of pathologists. Long-range studies on silicosis in its regions of prevalence by South African, Welsh, and American investigators have been fruitful. A very wide variety of toxemias of external cause have been studied. Not a few of these toxemias have developed in industry, including a greatly expanding drug industry. Nothing illustrates the hazards concerned better than the startling discovery in the early 1960's of a deadly action of the sedative drug thalidomide on limb development in the human embryo.

CANCER RESEARCH

Probably no field has been investigated more intensively than cancer, in part because of the large sums of money that have been made available through philanthropic and official funds for cancer research. The trend in the twentieth century, after the anatomical and theoretical studies of the nineteenth, has been toward experimental study of malignant tumors. This trend, inconspicuous at first, began with A. N. Hanau's successful transplantation, in Switzerland in 1889, of a carcinoma in the tissues of a rat. Leo Loeb in America in 1901 confirmed this result and went on in subsequent years to exhaustive studies of the transmission of malignant tumors, grafting, and the individuality of tissues. About the same time, the carcinogenic action of ionizing radiation in man was discovered through the observation of skin cancer in many radiologists, less than a decade after the discovery of x-rays. Later, x-rays were found to be a two-edged sword, destroying cancer as well as initiating it, and became an important element in the treatment of cancer. The mutational effect of ionizing radiation on cells, studied in pioneer investigations by H. J. Muller at Bloomington, Indiana, and others in the 1920's as a tool in genetic research, is under continual scrutiny in relation to the stimulation of cancer and leukemia.

Transplantation of tumors has since become one of the main procedures of cancer research. One of the early productive investigators was Carl Jensen in Copenhagen (1903 ff.), whose strain of transplantable mouse tumors was widely used. Studies on transplantable tumors, in the hands of E. E. Tyzzer in Boston

(1908 ff.), opened the way for a long series of investigations on heredity in cancer. Tyzzer, and subsequently Maud Slye in Chicago and C. C. Little in Michigan and Bar Harbor, Maine (1913 ff.), were among the most active protagonists of the theory of cancer heredity. Strains of mice, with a high incidence of spontaneous development of malignant tumors, particularly from the Jackson Memorial Laboratory, have been used as standard animals all over the world, and have been invaluable in studies of heredity and experimental therapy.

The possibility that cancer could be caused by a living virus has long had adherents. The hypothesis received strong support from the studies of Peyton Rous and his colleague J. B. Murphy on a transmissible sarcoma of fowls (1910 ff.). The etiological agent proved to be filterable. In 1913 Johannes Fibiger in Copenhagen reported an apparent etiological relationship between a parasite and carcinoma of the stomach in rats, an observation still of uncertain significance, but one that stimulated much research.

One of the most important of all developments in the field of carcinogenesis was the production by K. Yamagawa and K. Ichikawa in Tokyo, in 1915, of malignant tumors in the rabbit ear by inunction of coal tar. Much development in this field has taken place in recent years, mediated particularly by investigations by E. L. Kennaway and associates in England (1930 ff.) on the isolation from coal tar, or chemical synthesis, of pure hydrocarbons capable of inducing cancer on suitable application in animals. A variety of compounds of this class have since been used for the production of tumors for many types of research.

As indicated in the past few paragraphs, studies on the transplantation of tumors, heredity in tumor genesis, viral induction of tumors, and the production of cancer by chemically defined carcinogenic compounds have pushed cancer research forward rapidly. Throughout the same period increasing emphasis has been laid also on the relation of the body's hormones to tumor development. Among the many extended studies in this field, note should be made of the effect of estrogenic hormones on the induction and progress of breast tumors in mice, demonstrated by Lacassagne in Paris (1932) and others, and of the effect of male sex hormone on the progress of prostatic cancer in man and animals, shown by C. B. Huggins in Chicago (1941 ff.) and associates. A practical application of an understanding of the relations of cancer and female sex hormones is currently made in the science of "exfoliative cytology," initiated by G. N. Papanicolaou in New York (1933 ff.). The Papanicolaou test for cancer of the uterine cervix has become one of the commonest procedures in clinical pathology.

ADVANCES IN ORGAN PATHOLOGY

In the field of diseases of the cardiovascular system attention has been focussed particularly on the pathogenesis of atherosclerosis. Increasing weight has been given to the contention of N. Anitschkow in Leningrad, who attributed the basic lesion to excessive dietary intake of cholesterol (1913 ff.). Scouted at first, his hypothesis found much support in the experimental pathology of later years. Other important studies over the years have dealt with vascular hypertension, rheumatic fever, and the pathogenesis of coronary artery occlusion.

In the field of pulmonary pathology continuing attention has been devoted to types of pneumonia. Pneumococcus lobar pneumonia appears to have decreased with the passage of time and to have been supplanted by a number of virus inflammations of the lung. In this connection it is interesting to note that some of the most fruitful advances that have taken place in the field of genetics in recent years resulted from studies by O. T. Avery in New York and his associates on bacterial transformation induced by treating one type of pneumococcus with the desoxyribonucleic acid of a different type. These studies demonstrated the biological individuality of nucleic acids and improved understanding of the nature and action of genes. It should be noted in this connection that years previously (1910 ff.) T. H. Morgan of Columbia University had postulated an interchange of chromosomal material as a mechanism of mutation.

Another development in pulmonary pathology, observed in the experience of most pathologists, has been a notable increase in the incidence of primary bronchogenic carcinoma. The phenomenon has been correlated with irritants in inhaled air and particularly with tobacco smoke.

Knowledge of the pathogenesis of renal disease was in chaotic state at the end of the nineteenth century. New understanding was brought about by the studies of Franz Volhard and Theodor Fahr in Germany (1914 ff.). Out of these and other investigations of Bright's disease grew our current concepts of acute and chronic glomerular nephritis, those degenerative conditions now comprehended under the term nephrosis and the relation of vascular hypertension and arteriolar thickening to nephrosclerosis. Studies by Harry Goldblatt in Cleveland (1934 ff.) on the relation of the vascular state of the kidneys to vascular hypertension have been illuminating.

In the field of blood disease notable advances included the explanation of blood protein and corpuscle regeneration, the pathogenesis of pernicious anemia, the recognition of blood groups and understanding of incompatibility of bloods. The latter has been in large measure an outgrowth of the studies of Karl Landsteiner in Vienna (1900 ff.), to whom, primarily, we owe the modern classification of blood types. In later years (1940 ff.) in New York, Landsteiner and his associates, A. S. Wiener and P. Levine, brought about an understanding of the occasional incompatibilities of the blood of mother and offspring, with resultant erythrocyte destruction, due to the "Rh factor."

Modern treatment of the anemias, pernicious anemia in particular, stems from studies by G. H. Whipple in San Francisco and Rochester, New York, and his associates (1925 ff.) on the rôle of a liver factor in stimulating blood regeneration.

The supporting structures of the body and particularly its connective tissues have in general excited much less interest among pathologists than visceral lesions. However a new concept, that of "collagen disease," which was introduced by Paul Klemperer of New York and his associates (1942), helps in understanding the pathogenesis of a series of seemingly unrelated diseases, including rheumatic fever, rheumatoid arthritis, lupus erythematosus and periarteritis nodosa, ailments of presumably different etiology but with a factor in common in a disordered state of the collagenic matrix of connective tissue. The ultimate explanation of the pathogenesis of the underlying process will presumably depend on future biochemical studies.

In few fields have advances in the twentieth century been as great as in the pathology of disorders in the glands of internal secretion. Progress has been world-wide, following the early explorations of Brown-Séquard of Paris and other pioneers in the nineteenth century, to whose work reference is made in the final chapter of the book to which this brief account is appended. Anomalies due to excess or deficiency in the secretions of the separate lobes of the hypophysis, the thyroid and parathyroid glands, the pancreas, the adrenals and the sex organs have been studied in a wealth of detail. Epoch-marking investigations to which brief attention should be called include: the studies of

Harvey Cushing in Baltimore and Boston on tumors of the pituitary gland (1912 ff.); those of the chemist E. C. Kendall of the Mayo Foundation on the secretions of the thyroid gland (1915), which gave precision to subsequent pathological investigations of specific clinical thyroid disorders; the investigations of W. G. MacCallum in Baltimore on the rôle of the parathyroid glands in calcium metabolism and parathyroid tetany (1909); the discovery by Frederick Banting in Toronto and his associates of the rôle of the internal secretion of the pancreas in diabetes (1921 ff.); the studies of a large group of investigators all over the world who supplemented the earlier understanding of the adrenal-deficiency state long known as Addison's disease with new knowledge on water balance, salt retention, vascular hypertension, and sex gland associations; and finally the investigations of many observers, also world-wide in distribution, of anomalies of the sex glands themselves. The relation of specific structures within the glands to disease was well illustrated in the case of the pituitary gland and the pancreas. Cushing and others called attention to the clinical syndromes associated with basophil, acidophil or chromophobe cell adenomas of the former, and E. L. Opie in Baltimore (1901 ff.) focussed attention on a relation between degeneration of the islets of Langerhans in the pancreas and diabetes mellitus. Years later R. M. Wilder of the Mayo Clinic and others correlated the clinical state of hyperinsulinism with over-development and activity of these microscopic structures.

Improving knowledge of diseases of the central nervous system has stemmed in large measure from exact anatomical studies by the pioneer Italian neurohistologist Camillo Golgi (1883 ff.), and the Spanish histologists Santiago Ramón y Cajal (1889 ff.) and his pupil Pio del Rio Hortega (1918 ff.). Ramón y Cajal's classification of cells of the nervous system was an important stepping stone to a useful and systematic classification of brain tumors developed in later years by Harvey Cushing and Percival Bailey.

TEACHING OF PATHOLOGY

The foregoing has been a highly sketchy review, which at best can only indicate a few of the lines of endeavor and illustrate, through a minimum of special examples, trends that have been productive in pathological research.

The teaching of pathology in medical schools and hospitals

has kept up with advances in research. Progress throughout the world, which has made foreign travel desirable for the development of new contacts, has at the same time made it no longer indispensable, as it was in the late nineteenth century, when students from far-off lands journeyed to central Europe, and especially Germany and Vienna, for training in pathological anatomy. Teaching in the years of this century has tended more and more to be in the realm of functional pathology, with emphasis on correlations with physiology, on the one hand, and laboratory as well as general clinical medicine, with all their chemical, radiographic and electronic devices, on the other. Yet pathological anatomy remains fundamental in the teaching of pathology. A thoughtful American pathologist, H. T. Karsner, in reviewing the lives of great "career" professors of the past, noted that they were all first class morphologists, and added that modern teachers "are good experimentalists, but none ignores the importance of diseased form."

Inevitably classroom teaching has changed, with the introduction of more training in experimental pathology. A highly important trend has been a growing insistence on control in experiment and statistical reliability in conclusions.

The expansion of texts in pathology has more than kept pace with other advances in education. With increasing specialization, multiple authorship has become more common. In the ever growing multiplication of knowledge, improved compendia for assemblage, codification, and condensation of new information have become indispensable. An outstanding example is the well known *Handbuch der speziellen pathologischen Anatomie und Histologie* originally edited by the German pathologists Friedrich Henke, Otto Lubarsch and their associates (Berlin, 1924 ff.). A comparable set of authoritative compilations is to be found in the series of fascicles constituting the *Atlas of Tumor Pathology* more recently sponsored by the National Research Council and Armed Forces Institute of Pathology in the United States.

BRANCHES OF PATHOLOGY

In the development of pathology as an academic science fundamental to the understanding and practice of medicine, there has been less than logical correlation of human with general and comparative pathology. Institutes and journals for comparative pathology have existed for years in British and continental European centers, but they have been outside of the main stream of medical pathology or have been set up for a particular person, as in the case of the short-lived chair of comparative pathology created at Harvard University for Theobald Smith in 1896.

However, the subject has not been neglected, for it has been practiced on a larger scale in traditional veterinary pathology, in the pathological investigations that have become standard in zoölogical gardens all over the world, and everywhere in the field of plant pathology in departments of botany and agricultural experiment stations. In addition to this there has been a constant increase in the number of species of animals used by investigators of human pathology in experimentation. Thus, although the correlation of human and comparative pathology has not been as close as that of human and comparative anatomy, pertinent data in abundance for the correlations are available.

Veterinary pathology, noted above, with a wealth of schools, institutions, academic departments, special societies, and journals for its development, has become one of the major branches of pathology as a whole. In human pathology there has been a trend toward specialization in branches representative of the so-called specialties in medicine. Thus we find special societies, journals, and advanced texts in such individual fields as oral, dental, skin, and eye pathology, in all of which advance in knowledge has kept pace with progress in more general pathology.

For reasons that are readily apparent, in view of the magnitude of the field, pathology as related to tropical medicine has grown strikingly. A large part of the world's population lives in tropical regions and much of it in localities where sanitary conditions are bad and parasitic disease and its vectors widespread. The variety of ailments is reflected in such eponymic terms as Carrión's disease and Chagas' disease in South America, and in the massive campaigns to eradicate specific diseases and their vectors in Africa, South America, and the Orient. Schools and institutes of tropical medicine, in which the pathology of tropical diseases is heavily emphasized, have been established all over the world, in London, Liverpool, Hamburg, Calcutta, and San Juan, Puerto Rico, to mention but a few. To these might be added many institutes of more general purpose, but inevitably devoted in large measure, by virtue of location, to tropical disease pathology, such as the Gorgas Memorial Laboratory in Panama and the Oswaldo Cruz Institute in Brazil.

Among pathological specialties few have been of more immediate practical application than pathology in relation to forensic medicine. From time immemorial society has insisted on a definite designation of cause of death. For centuries this has meant some participation by the medical profession in the determination, which, to be sure, as often as not in the past, has been inadequate and faulty. With increasing precision in understanding, however, and especially through exact studies in pathology, medical pronouncement has gained greatly in accuracy. Cessation of life is often sudden, and even if gradual is often of obscure cause. It may come about through violence, or under unobserved circumstances. In either case, under modern conditions of society, the understanding of a pathologist has become indispensable in solution of the problem, and his findings are often followed up in judicial and legal processes.

Institutes of forensic medicine, in which a department of pathology is an important constituent, have been in existence in Europe for many years. Exact and illuminating studies, promoted by increasingly penetrating laboratory technics, have come out of them. More recently they have developed in America, a notable example being the organization inaugurated in the early 1960's in New York City. In America there has been a trend toward replacement of the old coroner system in medico-legal processes with a system of trained medical examiners, for which a background of pathology, including pathological anatomy and a wide range of clinical laboratory practice, is basic.

Contemporaneous with this has been a steady development of societies, texts, journals, and other media of communication for improvement in procedure in this pathological specialization.

SOCIETIES AND JOURNALS

Professional societies and journals play an increasingly important part in the rapidly developing expansion of knowledge and in the inevitably resultant separation of specialties from the general field. Throughout the world large and small national and local societies have been established for the promotion of understanding in pathology. City and provincial societies preceded national ones. The latter were organized at the turn of the century. In the old days of emphasis on pathological anatomy the Deutsche Pathologische Gesellschaft (1897) pioneered. The American Association of Pathologists and Bacteriologists was founded in 1901, and the Pathological Society of Great Britain and Ireland in 1906. In the middle years of the twentieth century there has been an increasing trend toward the establishment of international societies in pathology, as well as in other branches of medicine. The cultivation of a new type of pathology, so-called "geographic pathology," in which attention is focussed on difference in disease in different parts of the world, illustrates the trend.

Communication of knowledge and ideas has become the essence of progress in pathology, as in other sciences. A notable increase in journals devoted to pathology has occurred all over the world. Distinguished among them in the early years of the twentieth century, in addition to those mentioned previously (pp. 118 and 136), have been: in England, the *Journal of Pathology and Bacteriology* (1892) and the *British Journal of Experimental Pathology* (1920); in France, the *Journal de Physiologie et de Pathologie Général* (1899); in Germany, the *Frankfurter Zeitschrift für Pathologie* (1907); in Switzerland, the *Schweizerische Zeitschrift für allgemeine Pathologie und Bakteriologie* (1938); in Italy, the Genoese journal *Pathologica* (1908); in the Scandinavian countries the *Acta Pathologica et Microbiologica Scandinavica* (1924), published in Copenhagen; in Soviet Russia, an *Arkhiv* devoted to pathological anatomy and pathological physiology (1939), published in Moscow; and in the United States, the *American Journal of Pathology* (1925), the *Archives of Pathology* (1926), and the *American Journal of Clinical Pathology* (1931). The list is by no means exhaustive.

In addition to these, there are numerous journals devoted to branches of pathology, including comparative and veterinary pathology, and such special fields in human pathology as neuropathology, oral and dental pathology, and forensic pathology. The difficulty is no longer in finding media for publication, but in developing means of bringing new literature to the attention of those interested. For this purpose there are numerous abstract journals. At the time of writing, the latest compendium in this field, limited to names, titles, and journal references, is the mammoth *Current List of Medical Literature,* which has been sponsored coöperatively by the American Medical Association and the National Institutes of Health of the U. S. Public

Health Service. This has enabled a rapid scanning of the separate fields of medicine, leaving the major job of study and absorption to other media.

CLINICAL PATHOLOGY

Up to this point pathology has been treated as a unit, with due recognition of the fact that specialties exist within the parent discipline. Not to be ignored, however, is the fact that pathology as a principal medical discipline has long been divided, in the concept of practitioners of medicine, into two major categories, pathology without further definition, and clinical pathology, which is devoted largely to those laboratory procedures that have proven essential in the diagnosis of disease and estimation of its progress.

A recent author, W. D. Foster of Birmingham, England, has divided clinical pathology into morbid anatomy, chemical pathology, bacteriology and hematology, and in writing its history has emphasized its practical applications, making the pertinent observation that "although some of the great names in the history of pathology" figure in the story, "the majority of the heroes," i.e., in clinical pathology, "are not the great discoverers, but those men who took the new knowledge won by original workers and utilized it in everyday medicine."

The author of the present condensed appendix to an older book would leave the history of that large subject to Foster and others who have treated its details so competently. But in closing this brief direction of attention to twentieth-century progress in pathology as a whole, some mention of the apparent schism between general pathology and clinical pathology is necessary. The academic professor of pathology of the present century, who passed from the field of pathological anatomy to the methods of experimental pathology and an absorption in functional pathology, remained, for the bulk of that long period, more or less aloof from the laboratory problems confronting the internist or surgeon in his daily private or hospital practice.

Gradually, under one designation or another, men and women trained in the growing complexities of laboratory medicine developed departments of clinical pathology in hospitals and medical centers which in time became among the largest of all the hospital departments. In a sense, just as traditional pathology had formed a link between the basic anatomical sciences and clinical medicine, so clinical pathology forged an even more conspicuous chain between clinical medicine and the basic sciences of bacteriology, virology, hematology, biochemistry, and physiology. The huge number of functional and diagnostic tests made available in the development of those sciences in the twentieth century greatly enhanced the possibilities for precision in medical practice.

Withal, however, an essential unity has been evident in the two types of pathology, and in the middle years of the twentieth century increasing amalgamation has taken place in the two great institutions primarily concerned, i.e., the medical school and the hospital. The amalgamation has been fostered in part by a separate movement, the creation of large "medical centers" in which medical schools and associated hospitals are closely joined. The academic pathologist and the hospital or service pathologist each for his part recognizes an overlapping and dual responsibility, viz., in undergraduate and graduate teaching and in research, or, more definitively, the search for new knowledge. The system of teaching pathology prevalent today in many schools, particularly as seen in American schools, is patterned somewhat on procedures in other medical departments, involving a series of clerkships, rotating residencies, clinical-pathological conferences and other media drawing all pathology into closer relation with clinical medicine and surgery.

And this is perhaps a good place to leave the subject. The future of pathology as an academic and intellectual discipline is still to be worked out—a trite statement, to be sure, for it is true of all sciences. But there is little reason to foresee any true schism within the major field. Rather, a new definition of pathology is needed.

Index of Personal Names

Abbe, Ernst, 129
Abernethy, John, 92
Adami, J. G., 174
Addison, Thomas, 97-9, 140
Addison, William, 100
Aëtius of Amida, 16, 24
Agramonte, Aristides, 155
Albinus, Bernard Siegfried, 72
Alexander of Tralles, 24, 26
Andral, Gabriel, 83, 84, 94, 105, 108,
    121, 166
Andrews, C. H., 175
Anitschkow, N., 179
Archigenes of Apameia, 16, 17, 24
Archilochus, 8
Aretaeus of Cappadocia, 16-7
Aristotle, 9, 26
Arnold, Julius, 136-7
Aschoff, Ludwig, 168, 174
Asclepiades of Bithynia, 12, 13
Astruc, Jean, 65-6
Athenaeus of Cilicia, 12
Athothis, 2
Auenbrugger, Leopold, 77, 103
Avenzoar, 26, 44
Avery, O. T., 179
Avicenna, 26, 27, 30, 45

Baglivi, Giorgio, 58, 59
Bailey, Percival, 181
Baillie, Matthew, 64, 70, 93-4
Banting, Frederick, 181
Bartholin, Thomas, 52-3
Bartolomeo da Varignana, 27, 28
Basedow, Karl von, 163
Bassi, Agostino, 144
Bauhin, Caspar, 44
Bayle, Gaspard-Laurent, 80-1, 82

Béclard, Pierre-Augustin, 80, 85
Behring, Emil von, 151
Benedetti, Alessandro, 35, 44, 48
Benivieni, Antonio, 26, 31-5, 38, 42
Benivieni, Geronimo, 31-2, 61
Bennett, John Hughes, 100, 120
Berengario da Carpi, Giacomo, 35-6
Bernard, Claude, 139, 162
Bichat, Marie-François-Xavier, 72, 77,
    78-80, 81, 85, 102, 129
Biermayer, Lorenz, 104
Biermer, Anton, 140
Billroth, Theodor, 113, 125, 132
Bizzozero, Giulio, 137
Blankaart, Steven, 62
Böhmer, F., 131
Blum, J., 131
Boccaccio, Giovanni, 142
Böhmer, F., 131
Boerhaave, Hermann, 51, 73-4, 102
Bollinger, Otto, 137
Bonet, Théophile, 59-62, 68
Bonn, Andreas, 72
Bontius, Jacob, 50
Bordet, Jules, 154
Bordeu, Théophile de, 163
Bostock, John, 97
Bouillaud, Jean-Baptiste, 87-8, 94
Bouwmanno, Maximiliano, 64
Bretonneau, Pierre, 82
Bright, Richard, 40, 95-7, 99, 166
Broca, Paul, 88
Brodie, Sir Benjamin, 139
Broussais, François-Joseph-Victor, 75,
    83-4
Brown, John, 74-5, 83
Brown-Séquard, Charles-Édouard, 139,
    162-3, 180

Gull, Sir William, 139, 163
Guy, Thomas, 95
Guy de Chauliac, 29-30

Haën, Anton de, 73, 102-3
Haller, Albrecht von, 72, 74
Hanau, A. N., 177
Hannover, Adolf, 130
Hansen, Armauer, 245
Harrison, R. G., 173
Harvey, William, 35, 46, 48, 64, 156, 157
Hayem, Georges, 137
Heberden, William, 89
Hebra, Ferdinand von, 105
Heiberg, Hjalmar, 133
Heidenhain, Rudolf, 130, 134, 161
Heister, Lorenz, 41
Helmont, Jean-Baptiste van, 12, 46, 51
Henke, Friedrich, 182
Henle, Jacob, 115, 116, 144, 147
Henri de Mondeville, 27, 29-30
Hermann, F., 131
Herophilus, 9-10, 11
Heschl, Richard, 111, 112
Hevesy, Georg von, 173
Hippocrates, 5-6, 13, 17, 18, 21, 24, 26, 43, 57
His, Wilhelm, 130
Hodgkin, Thomas, 99
Hodgson, Joseph, 70, 95, 99
Hoffmann, Erich, 151
Hoffmann, Friedrich, 72
Holmes, Oliver Wendell, 112, 143
Home, Everard, 92
Hope, James, 94
Hopkins, F. Gowland, 176
Hoppe-Seyler, Felix, 166
Horner, William Edmonds, 101
Huggins, C. B., 178
Hunter, John, 37, 72, 88, 90-3, 108, 109, 152, 158
Hunter, William, 90, 93
Hutchinson, Sir Jonathan, 139-40
Hutin, 137
Hyrtl, Josef, 105

Ichikawa, K., 178
Israel, Oscar, 137

Jenner, Edward, 92, 93, 113, 143
Jensen, Carl, 177
Joubertus, Laurent, 48

Kaiserling, Carl, 131
Karsner, H. T., 182
Kartulis, Stephanos, 150
Kendall, E. C., 181
Kennaway, E. L., 178
Kentmann, Johann, 44
Kerkring, Theodore, 62
Kircher, Athanasius, 58
Kitasato, Shibasaburo, 150, 151
Klebs, Edwin, 112, 126, 130, 132-3, 138, 149, 150
Klemperer, Paul, 180
Koch, Robert, 124, 133, 147-9, 150, 151, 161
Kocher, Theodor, 163
Kolisko, Alexander, 111-2
Kraus, Rudolf, 152
Kundrat, Hanns, 111, 112

Lacassagne, A. M. B., 178
Laënnec, René-Théophile-Hyacinthe, 77, 80, 81-2, 105, 110, 124
Laidlaw, P. P., 175
Lamzweerde, Joh. Baptista, 50
Lancisi, Giovanni Maria, 37, 58, 67
Landsteiner, Karl, 180
Laveran, Alphonse, 154
Lazear, Jesse W., 155
Lebert, Hermann, 117, 134, 172
Le Dran, Henri François, 65
Leeuwenhoek, Antonj van, 58
Leonardo da Vinci, 29
Leonides of Alexandria, 24
Levine, P., 180
Liebig, Justus von, 166
Lieutaud, Joseph, 66-7
Lister, Lord Joseph, 146
Lister, Joseph Jackson, 129
Little, C. C., 178
Lobstein, Johann Martin, 84-5, 105, 109
Loeb, Leo, 177
Löffler, Friedrich, 149, 150
Louis, Antoine, 65
Louis, Pierre-Charles-Alexandre, 82-3
Lower, Richard, 61, 157
Lubarsch, Otto, 182

Index of Subjects

Abscess, 4, 8, 13-4, 30, 35, 40, 48, 120-1
  brain, 53
  tonsillar, 43
Acidosis, 51, 167
Acromegaly, 138, 162
Actinomycosis, 137, 144
Addison's disease, 98, 181
Adenomyoma, 132
Agglutination, 152
Albuminuria, 96
Alexandrian school, 4, 9-11, 13, 15
Alkalosis, 51
Allergic inflammation, 174
Amyloidosis, 110, 111, 123
Anaphylaxis, 154
Anasarca, 17, 19, 41, 96
Anemia, 165, 180
  primary, 84, 98, 140
  secondary, 84
Aneurysm, 2, 41, 45, 55, 69-70, 72, 95
  aortic, 37, 55, 57, 61, 64, 69-70, 78, 82, 95, 101
Angina pectoris, 89, 93, 162
Animism, 73
Anthracosis, 4, 80
Anthrax, 30, 71, 144-5, 146, 147
Antibodies, 154, 173, 174
Antitoxins, 151-2
Aortic insufficiency, 48, 65, 99-100
Aortitis, syphilitic, 70, 87
Aphasia, 88, 138
Apoplexy, 43, 44, 53, 54, 56, 58, 69
Appendicitis, 13, 41
Arabian medicine, 25-7
Archaeus, 46
Arterio-capillary fibrosis, 139
Arteriosclerosis, 4, 55, 58, 72, 93, 137, 139
Arthritis, 11

rheumatoid, 180
Arthritis deformans, 4
Ascites, 11, 17, 19, 24, 61, 71, 96, 157
Asepsis, 45, 146
Aspergillosis, 144
Assyrians, 5
Atelectasis, 99
Atherosclerosis, 179
Atra bilis, 7, 13, 18, 22, 23, 46

Babylonians, 5
Bacteriolysis, 152
Beri-beri, 50
Black bile (see also atra bilis), 6, 20, 22-3
Blastema, 107, 110, 116
Blood, circulation of, 47-8
Blood chemistry, 84, 97, 167
Bones, pathology of, 64, 72, 132, 139
Boniface VIII, Bull of, 28
Bright's disease (see also nephritis), 28, 96, 164, 179
Bronchiectasis, 81
Bronchitis, 21, 70
  fibrinous, 43, 50
Brucellosis, 175
Brunonism, 74-5
Burns, 45

Calcification, 65, 111, 274
Calculi, 46, 50, 64
  biliary (see gallstones)
  sublingual, 41
  urinary, 14, 21, 40, 50, 53, 58, 61, 64, 71, 72
Cancer (see also carcinoma), 7, 23, 29-30, 41, 45, 46, 50, 65, 81-2, 87, 94, 109, 124-5
  and hormones, 178
  and viruses, 178

CATALOGUE OF DOVER BOOKS

Books Explaining Science and Mathematics

WHAT IS SCIENCE?, N. Campbell. The role of experiment and measurement, the function of mathematics, the nature of scientific laws, the difference between laws and theories, the limitations of science, and many similarly provocative topics are treated clearly and without technicalities by an eminent scientist. "Still an excellent introduction to scientific philosophy," H. Margenau in PHYSICS TODAY. "A first-rate primer . . . deserves a wide audience," SCIENTIFIC AMERICAN. 192pp. 5⅜ x 8.   S43 Paperbound **$1.25**

THE NATURE OF PHYSICAL THEORY, P. W. Bridgman. A Nobel Laureate's clear, non-technical lectures on difficulties and paradoxes connected with frontier research on the physical sciences. Concerned with such central concepts as thought, logic, mathematics, relativity, probability, wave mechanics, etc. he analyzes the contributions of such men as Newton, Einstein, Bohr, Heisenberg, and many others. "Lucid and entertaining . . . recommended to anyone who wants to get some insight into current philosophies of science," THE NEW PHILOSOPHY. Index. xi + 138pp. 5⅜ x 8.   S33 Paperbound **$1.25**

EXPERIMENT AND THEORY IN PHYSICS, Max Born. A Nobel Laureate examines the nature of experiment and theory in theoretical physics and analyzes the advances made by the great physicists of our day: Heisenberg, Einstein, Bohr, Planck, Dirac, and others. The actual process of creation is detailed step-by-step by one who participated. A fine examination of the scientific method at work. 44pp. 5⅜ x 8.   S308 Paperbound **75¢**

THE PSYCHOLOGY OF INVENTION IN THE MATHEMATICAL FIELD, J. Hadamard. The reports of such men as Descartes, Pascal, Einstein, Poincaré, and others are considered in this investigation of the method of idea-creation in mathematics and other sciences and the thinking process in general. How do ideas originate? What is the role of the unconscious? What is Poincaré's forgetting hypothesis? are some of the fascinating questions treated. A penetrating analysis of Einstein's thought processes concludes the book. xiii + 145pp. 5⅜ x 8.   T107 Paperbound **$1.25**

THE NATURE OF LIGHT AND COLOUR IN THE OPEN AIR, M. Minnaert. Why are shadows sometimes blue, sometimes green, or other colors depending on the light and surroundings? What causes mirages? Why do multiple suns and moons appear in the sky? Professor Minnaert explains these unusual phenomena and hundreds of others in simple, easy-to-understand terms based on optical laws and the properties of light and color. No mathematics is required but artists, scientists, students, and everyone fascinated by these "tricks" of nature will find thousands of useful and amazing pieces of information. Hundreds of observational experiments are suggested which require no special equipment. 200 illustrations; 42 photos. xvi + 362pp. 5⅜ x 8.   T196 Paperbound **$2.00**

THE UNIVERSE OF LIGHT, W. Bragg. Sir William Bragg, Nobel Laureate and great modern physicist, is also well known for his powers of clear exposition. Here he analyzes all aspects of light for the layman: lenses, reflection, refraction, the optics of vision, x-rays, the photoelectric effect, etc. He tells you what causes the color of spectra, rainbows, and soap bubbles, how magic mirrors work, and much more. Dozens of simple experiments are described. Preface. Index. 199 line drawings and photographs, including 2 full-page color plates. x + 283pp. 5⅜ x 8.   T538 Paperbound **$1.85**

SOAP-BUBBLES: THEIR COLOURS AND THE FORCES THAT MOULD THEM, C. V. Boys. For continuing popularity and validity as scientific primer, few books can match this volume of easily-followed experiments, explanations. Lucid exposition of complexities of liquid films, surface tension and related phenomena, bubbles' reaction to heat, motion, music, magnetic fields. Experiments with capillary attraction, soap bubbles on frames, composite bubbles, liquid cylinders and jets, bubbles other than soap, etc. Wonderful introduction to scientific method, natural laws that have many ramifications in areas of modern physics. Only complete edition in print. New Introduction by S. Z. Lewin, New York University. 83 illustrations; 1 full-page color plate. xii + 190pp. 5⅜ x 8½.   T542 Paperbound **95¢**

THE STORY OF X-RAYS FROM RONTGEN TO ISOTOPES, A. R. Bleich, M.D. This book, by a member of the American College of Radiology, gives the scientific explanation of x-rays, their applications in medicine, industry and art, and their danger (and that of atmospheric radiation) to the individual and the species. You learn how radiation therapy is applied against cancer, how x-rays diagnose heart disease and other ailments, how they are used to examine mummies for information on diseases of early societies, and industrial materials for hidden weaknesses. 54 illustrations show x-rays of flowers, bones, stomach, gears with flaws, etc. 1st publication. Index. xix + 186pp. 5⅜ x 8. T622 Paperbound **$1.50**

SPINNING TOPS AND GYROSCOPIC MOTION, John Perry. A classic elementary text of the dynamics of rotation — the behavior and use of rotating bodies such as gyroscopes and tops. In simple, everyday English you are shown how quasi-rigidity is induced in discs of paper, smoke rings, chains, etc., by rapid motions; why a gyrostat falls and why a top rises; precession; how the earth's motion affects climate; and many other phenomena. Appendix on practical use of gyroscopes. 62 figures. 128pp. 5⅜ x 8. T416 Paperbound **$1.25**

SNOW CRYSTALS, W. A. Bentley, M. J. Humphreys. For almost 50 years W. A. Bentley photographed snow flakes in his laboratory in Jericho, Vermont; in 1931 the American Meteorological Society gathered together the best of his work, some 2400 photographs of snow flakes, plus a few ice flowers, windowpane frosts, dew, frozen rain, and other ice formations. Pictures were selected for beauty and scientific value. A very valuable work to anyone in meteorology, cryology; most interesting to layman; extremely useful for artist who wants beautiful, crystalline designs. All copyright free. Unabridged reprint of 1931 edition. 2453 illustrations. 227pp. 8 x 10½. T287 Paperbound **$3.00**

A DOVER SCIENCE SAMPLER, edited by George Barkin. A collection of brief, non-technical passages from 44 Dover Books Explaining Science for the enjoyment of the science-minded browser. Includes work of Bertrand Russell, Poincaré, Laplace, Max Born, Galileo, Newton; material on physics, mathematics, metallurgy, anatomy, astronomy, chemistry, etc. You will be fascinated by Martin Gardner's analysis of the sincere pseudo-scientist, Moritz's account of Newton's absentmindedness, Bernard's examples of human vivisection, etc. Illustrations from the Diderot Pictorial Encyclopedia and De Re Metallica. 64 pages. **FREE**

THE STORY OF ATOMIC THEORY AND ATOMIC ENERGY, J. G. Feinberg. A broader approach to subject of nuclear energy and its cultural implications than any other similar source. Very readable, informal, completely non-technical text. Begins with first atomic theory, 600 B.C. and carries you through the work of Mendelejeff, Röntgen, Madame Curie, to Einstein's equation and the A-bomb. New chapter goes through thermonuclear fission, binding energy, other events up to 1959. Radioactive decay and radiation hazards, future benefits, work of Bohr, moderns, hundreds more topics. "Deserves special mention . . . not only authoritative but thoroughly popular in the best sense of the word," Saturday Review. Formerly, "The Atom Story." Expanded with new chapter. Three appendixes. Index. 34 illustrations. vii + 243pp. 5⅜ x 8. T625 Paperbound **$1.60**

THE STRANGE STORY OF THE QUANTUM, AN ACCOUNT FOR THE GENERAL READER OF THE GROWTH OF IDEAS UNDERLYING OUR PRESENT ATOMIC KNOWLEDGE, B. Hoffmann. Presents lucidly and expertly, with barest amount of mathematics, the problems and theories which led to modern quantum physics. Dr. Hoffmann begins with the closing years of the 19th century, when certain trifling discrepancies were noticed, and with illuminating analogies and examples takes you through the brilliant concepts of Planck, Einstein, Pauli, Broglie, Bohr, Schroedinger, Heisenberg, Dirac, Sommerfeld, Feynman, etc. This edition includes a new, long postscript carrying the story through 1958. "Of the books attempting an account of the history and contents of our modern atomic physics which have come to my attention, this is the best," H. Margenau, Yale University, in "American Journal of Physics." 32 tables and line illustrations. Index. 275pp. 5⅜ x 8. T518 Paperbound **$1.50**

SPACE AND TIME, E. Borel. Written by a versatile mathematician of world renown with his customary lucidity and precision, this introduction to relativity for the layman presents scores of examples, analogies, and illustrations that open up new ways of thinking about space and time. It covers abstract geometry and geographical maps, continuity and topology, the propagation of light, the special theory of relativity, the general theory of relativity, theoretical researches, and much more. Mathematical notes. 2 Indexes. 4 Appendices. 15 figures. xvi + 243pp. 5⅜ x 8. T592 Paperbound **$1.75**

FROM EUCLID TO EDDINGTON: A STUDY OF THE CONCEPTIONS OF THE EXTERNAL WORLD, Sir Edmund Whittaker. A foremost British scientist traces the development of theories of natural philosophy from the western rediscovery of Euclid to Eddington, Einstein, Dirac, etc. The inadequacy of classical physics is contrasted with present day attempts to understand the physical world through relativity, non-Euclidean geometry, space curvature, wave mechanics, etc. 5 major divisions of examination: Space; Time and Movement; the Concepts of Classical Physics; the Concepts of Quantum Mechanics; the Eddington Universe 212pp. 5⅜ x 8. T491 Paperbound **$1.35**

Nature, Biology,

NATURE RECREATION: Group Guidance for the Out-of-doors, William Gould Vinal. Intended for both the uninitiated nature instructor and the education student on the college level, this complete "how-to" program surveys the entire area of nature education for the young. Philosophy of nature recreation; requirements, responsibilities, important information for group leaders; nature games; suggested group projects; conducting meetings and getting discussions started; etc. Scores of immediately applicable teaching aids, plus completely updated sources of information, pamphlets, field guides, recordings, etc. Bibliography. 74 photographs. + 310pp. 5⅜ x 8½.　　　　　　　　　　　　T1015 Paperbound **$1.75**

HOW TO KNOW THE WILD FLOWERS, Mrs. William Starr Dana. Classic nature book that has introduced thousands to wonders of American wild flowers. Color-season principle of organ- ization is easy to use, even by those with no botanical training, and the genial, refreshing discussions of history, folklore, uses of over 1,000 native and escape flowers, foliage plants are informative as well as fun to read. Over 170 full-page plates, collected from several editions, may be colored in to make permanent records of finds. Revised to conform with 1950 edition of Gray's Manual of Botany. xlii + 438pp. 5⅜ x 8½.　　T332 Paperbound **$2.00**

HOW TO KNOW THE FERNS, F. T. Parsons. Ferns, among our most lovely native plants, are all too little known. This classic of nature lore will enable the layman to identify almost any American fern he may come across. After an introduction on the structure and life of ferns, the 57 most important ferns are fully pictured and described (arranged upon a simple identifi- cation key). Index of Latin and English names. 61 illustrations and 42 full-page plates. xiv + 215pp. 5⅜ x 8.　　　　　　　　　　　　　　　　　　　T740 Paperbound **$1.35**

MANUAL OF THE TREES OF NORTH AMERICA, Charles Sprague Sargent. Still unsurpassed as most comprehensive, reliable study of North American tree characteristics, precise locations and distribution. By dean of American dendrologists. Every tree native to U.S., Canada, Alaska, 185 genera, 717 species, described in detail—leaves, flowers, fruit, winterbuds, bark, wood, growth habits etc. plus discussion of varieties and local variants, immaturity variations. Over 100 keys, including unusual 11-page analytical key to genera, aid in identi- fication. 783 clear illustrations of flowers, fruit, leaves. An unmatched permanent reference work for all nature lovers. Second enlarged (1926) edition. Synopsis of families. Analytical key to genera. Glossary of technical terms. Index. 783 illustrations, 1 map. Two volumes. Total of 982pp. 5⅜ x 8.　　　　　　　　　　　　　　T277 Vol. I Paperbound **$2.25**
　　　　　　　　　　　　　　　　　　　　　　　　　T278 Vol. II Paperbound **$2.25**
　　　　　　　　　　　　　　　　　　　　　　　　　The set **$4.50**

TREES OF THE EASTERN AND CENTRAL UNITED STATES AND CANADA, W. M. Harlow. A revised edition of a standard middle-level guide to native trees and important escapes. More than 140 trees are described in detail, and illustrated with more than 600 drawings and photo- graphs. Supplementary keys will enable the careful reader to identify almost any tree he might encounter. xiii + 288pp. 5⅜ x 8.　　　　　　　　　T395 Paperbound **$1.35**

GUIDE TO SOUTHERN TREES, Ellwood S. Harrar and J. George Harrar. All the essential in- formation about trees indigenous to the South, in an extremely handy format. Introductory essay on methods of tree classification and study, nomenclature, chief divisions of Southern trees, etc. Approximately 100 keys and synopses allow for swift, accurate identification of trees. Numerous excellent illustrations, non-technical text make this a useful book for teachers of biology or natural science, nature lovers, amateur naturalists. Revised 1962 edition. Index. Bibliography. Glossary of technical terms. 920 illustrations; 201 full-page plates. ix + 709pp. 4⅝ x 6⅜.　　　　　　　　　　　　　　T945 Paperbound **$2.35**

FRUIT KEY AND TWIG KEY TO TREES AND SHRUBS, W. M. Harlow. Bound together in one volume for the first time, these handy and accurate keys to fruit and twig identification are the only guides of their sort with photographs (up to 3 times natural size). "Fruit Key": Key to over 120 different deciduous and evergreen fruits. 139 photographs and 11 line drawings. Synoptic summary of fruit types. Bibliography. 2 Indexes (common and scientific names). "Twig Key": Key to over 160 different twigs and buds. 173 photographs. Glossary of technical terms. Bibli- ography. 2 Indexes (common and scientific names). Two volumes bound as one. Total of xvii + 126pp. 5⅝ x 8⅜.　　　　　　　　　　　　　　　　T511 Paperbound **$1.25**

INSECT LIFE AND INSECT NATURAL HISTORY, S. W. Frost. A work emphasizing habits, social life, and ecological relations of insects, rather than more academic aspects of classification and morphology. Prof. Frost's enthusiasm and knowledge are everywhere evident as he dis- cusses insect associations and specialized habits like leaf-rolling, leaf-mining, and case- making, the gall insects, the boring insects, aquatic insects, etc. He examines all sorts of matters not usually covered in general works, such as: insects as human food, insect music and musicians, insect response to electric and radio waves, use of insects in art and literature. The admirably executed purpose of this book, which covers the middle ground between ele- mentary treatment and scholarly monographs, is to excite the reader to observe for himself. Over 700 illustrations. Extensive bibliography. x + 524pp. 5⅜ x 8.　　T517 Paperbound **$2.50**

CATALOGUE OF DOVER BOOKS

COMMON SPIDERS OF THE UNITED STATES, J. H. Emerton. Here is a nature hobby you can pursue right in your own cellar! Only non-technical, but thorough, reliable guide to spiders for the layman. Over 200 spiders from all parts of the country, arranged by scientific classification, are identified by shape and color, number of eyes, habitat and range, habits, etc. Full text, 501 line drawings and photographs, and valuable introduction explain webs, poisons, threads, capturing and preserving spiders, etc. Index. New synoptic key by S. W. Frost. xxiv + 225pp. 5⅜ x 8. **T223 Paperbound $1.45**

THE LIFE STORY OF THE FISH: HIS MANNERS AND MORALS, Brian Curtis. A comprehensive, non-technical survey of just about everything worth knowing about fish. Written for the aquarist, the angler, and the layman with an inquisitive mind, the text covers such topics as evolution, external covering and protective coloration, physics and physiology of vision, maintenance of equilibrium, function of the lateral line canal for auditory and temperature senses, nervous system, function of the air bladder, reproductive system and methods—courtship, mating, spawning, care of young—and many more. Also sections on game fish, the problems of conservation and a fascinating chapter on fish curiosities. "Clear, simple language . . . excellent judgment in choice of subjects . . . delightful sense of humor," New York Times. Revised (1949) edition. Index. Bibliography of 72 items. 6 full-page photographic plates. xii + 284pp. 5⅜ x 8. **T929 Paperbound $1.65**

BATS, Glover Morrill Allen. The most comprehensive study of bats as a life-form by the world's foremost authority. A thorough summary of just about everything known about this fascinating and mysterious flying mammal, including its unique location sense, hibernation and cycles, its habitats and distribution, its wing structure and flying habits, and its relationship to man in the long history of folklore and superstition. Written on a middle-level, the book can be profitably studied by a trained zoologist and thoroughly enjoyed by the layman. "An absorbing text with excellent illustrations. Bats should have more friends and fewer thoughtless detractors as a result of the publication of this volume," William Beebe, Books. Extensive bibliography. 57 photographs and illustrations. x + 368pp. 5⅜ x 8½. **T984 Paperbound $2.00**

BIRDS AND THEIR ATTRIBUTES, Glover Morrill Allen. A fine general introduction to birds as living organisms, especially valuable because of emphasis on structure, physiology, habits, behavior. Discusses relationship of bird to man, early attempts at scientific ornithology, feathers and coloration, skeletal structure including bills, legs and feet, wings. Also food habits, evolution and present distribution, feeding and nest-building, still unsolved questions of migrations and location sense, many more similar topics. Final chapter on classification, nomenclature. A good popular-level summary for the biologist; a first-rate introduction for the layman. Reprint of 1925 edition. References and index. 51 illustrations. viii + 338pp. 5⅜ x 8½. **T957 Paperbound $1.85**

LIFE HISTORIES OF NORTH AMERICAN BIRDS, Arthur Cleveland Bent. Bent's monumental series of books on North American birds, prepared and published under auspices of Smithsonian Institute, is the definitive coverage of the subject, the most-used single source of information. Now the entire set is to be made available by Dover in inexpensive editions. This encyclopedic collection of detailed, specific observations utilizes reports of hundreds of contemporary observers, writings of such naturalists as Audubon, Burroughs, William Brewster, as well as author's own extensive investigations. Contains literally everything known about life history of each bird considered: nesting, eggs, plumage, distribution and migration, voice, enemies, courtship, etc. These not over-technical works are musts for ornithologists, conservationists, amateur naturalists, anyone seriously interested in American birds.

BIRDS OF PREY. More than 100 subspecies of hawks, falcons, eagles, buzzards, condors and owls, from the common barn owl to the extinct caracara of Guadaloupe Island. 400 photographs. Two volume set. Index for each volume. Bibliographies of 403, 520 items. 197 full-page plates. Total of 907pp. 5⅜ x 8½.
Vol. I **T931 Paperbound $2.50**
Vol. II **T932 Paperbound $2.50**

WILD FOWL. Ducks, geese, swans, and tree ducks—73 different subspecies. Two volume set. Index for each volume. Bibliographies of 124, 144 items. 106 full-page plates. Total of 685pp. 5⅜ x 8½.
Vol. I **T285 Paperbound $2.50**
Vol. II **T286 Paperbound $2.50**

SHORE BIRDS. 81 varieties (sandpipers, woodcocks, plovers, snipes, phalaropes, curlews, oyster catchers, etc.). More than 200 photographs of eggs, nesting sites, adult and young of important species. Two volume set. Index for each volume. Bibliographies of 261, 188 items. 121 full-page plates. Total of 860pp. 5⅜ x 8½.
Vol. I **T933 Paperbound $2.35**
Vol. II **T934 Paperbound $2.35**

THE LIFE OF PASTEUR, R. Vallery-Radot. 13th edition of this definitive biography, cited in Encyclopaedia Britannica. Authoritative, scholarly, well-documented with contemporary quotes, observations; gives complete picture of Pasteur's personal life; especially thorough presentation of scientific activities with silkworms, fermentation, hydrophobia, inoculation, etc. Introduction by Sir William Osler. Index. 505pp. 5⅜ x 8. **T632 Paperbound $2.00**

Puzzles, Mathematical Recreations

SYMBOLIC LOGIC and THE GAME OF LOGIC, Lewis Carroll. "Symbolic Logic" is not concerned with modern symbolic logic, but is instead a collection of over 380 problems posed with charm and imagination, using the syllogism, and a fascinating diagrammatic method of drawing conclusions. In "The Game of Logic" Carroll's whimsical imagination devises a logical game played with 2 diagrams and counters (included) to manipulate hundreds of tricky syllogisms. The final section, "Hit or Miss" is a lagniappe of 101 additional puzzles in the delightful Carroll manner. Until this reprint edition, both of these books were rarities costing up to $15 each. Symbolic Logic: Index. xxxi + 199pp. The Game of Logic: 96pp. 2 vols. bound as one. 5⅜ x 8.   T492 Paperbound **$1.75**

PILLOW PROBLEMS and A TANGLED TALE, Lewis Carroll. One of the rarest of all Carroll's works, "Pillow Problems" contains 72 original math puzzles, all typically ingenious. Particularly fascinating are Carroll's answers which remain exactly as he thought them out, reflecting his actual mental process. The problems in "A Tangled Tale" are in story form, originally appearing as a monthly magazine serial. Carroll not only gives the solutions, but uses answers sent in by readers to discuss wrong approaches and misleading paths, and grades them for insight. Both of these books were rarities until this edition, "Pillow Problems" costing up to $25, and "A Tangled Tale" $15. Pillow Problems: Preface and Introduction by Lewis Carroll. xx + 109pp. A Tangled Tale: 6 illustrations. 152pp. Two vols. bound as one. 5⅜ x 8.   T493 Paperbound **$1.50**

AMUSEMENTS IN MATHEMATICS, Henry Ernest Dudeney. The foremost British originator of mathematical puzzles is always intriguing, witty, and paradoxical in this classic, one of the largest collections of mathematical amusements. More than 430 puzzles, problems, and paradoxes. Mazes and games, problems on number manipulation, unicursal and other route problems, puzzles on measuring, weighing, packing, age, kinship, chessboards, joiners', crossing river, plane figure dissection, and many others. Solutions. More than 450 illustrations. vii +. 258pp. 5⅜ x 8.   T473 Paperbound **$1.25**

THE CANTERBURY PUZZLES, Henry Dudeney. Chaucer's pilgrims set one another problems in story form. Also Adventures of the Puzzle Club, the Strange Escape of the King's Jester, the Monks of Riddlewell, the Squire's Christmas Puzzle Party, and others. All puzzles are original, based on dissecting plane figures, arithmetic, algebra, elementary calculus and other branches of mathematics, and purely logical ingenuity. "The limit of ingenuity and intricacy," The Observer. Over 110 puzzles. Full Solutions. 150 illustrations. vii + 225pp. 5⅜ x 8.   T474 Paperbound **$1.25**

MATHEMATICAL EXCURSIONS, H. A. Merrill. Even if you hardly remember your high school math, you'll enjoy the 90 stimulating problems contained in this book and you will come to understand a great many mathematical principles with surprisingly little effort. Many useful shortcuts and diversions not generally known are included: division by inspection, Russian peasant multiplication, memory systems for pi, building odd and even magic squares, square roots by geometry, dyadic systems, and many more. Solutions to difficult problems. 50 illustrations. 145pp. 5⅜ x 8.   T350 Paperbound **$1.00**

MAGIC SQUARES AND CUBES, W. S. Andrews. Only book-length treatment in English, a thorough non-technical description and analysis. Here are nasik, overlapping, pandiagonal, serrated squares; magic circles, cubes, spheres, rhombuses. Try your hand at 4-dimensional magical figures! Much unusual folklore and tradition included. High school algebra is sufficient. 754 diagrams and illustrations. viii + 419pp. 5⅜ x 8.   T658 Paperbound **$1.85**

CALIBAN'S PROBLEM BOOK: MATHEMATICAL, INFERENTIAL AND CRYPTOGRAPHIC PUZZLES, H. Phillips (Caliban), S. T. Shovelton, G. S. Marshall. 105 ingenious problems by the greatest living creator of puzzles on logic and inference. Rigorous, modern, piquant; reflecting their author's unusual personality, these intermediate and advanced puzzles all involve the ability to reason clearly through complex situations; some call for mathematical knowledge, ranging from algebra to number theory. Solutions. xi + 180pp. 5⅜ x 8.   T736 Paperbound **$1.25**

MATHEMATICAL PUZZLES FOR BEGINNERS AND ENTHUSIASTS, G. Mott-Smith. 188 mathematical puzzles based on algebra, dissection of plane figures, permutations, and probability, that will test and improve your powers of inference and interpretation. The Odic Force, The Spider's Cousin, Ellipse Drawing, theory and strategy of card and board games like tit-tat-toe, go moku, salvo, and many others. 100 pages of detailed mathematical explanations. Appendix of primes, square roots, etc. 135 illustrations. 2nd revised edition. 248pp. 5⅜ x 8.   T198 Paperbound **$1.00**

MATHEMAGIC, MAGIC PUZZLES, AND GAMES WITH NUMBERS, R. V. Heath. More than 60 new puzzles and stunts based on the properties of numbers. Easy techniques for multiplying large numbers mentally, revealing hidden numbers magically, finding the date of any day in any year, and dozens more. Over 30 pages devoted to magic squares, triangles, cubes, circles, etc. Edited by J. S. Meyer. 76 illustrations. 128pp. 5⅜ x 8.   T110 Paperbound **$1.00**

CATALOGUE OF DOVER BOOKS

THE BOOK OF MODERN PUZZLES, G. L. Kaufman. A completely new series of puzzles as fascinating as crossword and deduction puzzles but based upon different principles and techniques. Simple 2-minute teasers, word labyrinths, design and pattern puzzles, logic and observation puzzles — over 150 braincrackers. Answers to all problems. 116 illustrations. 192pp. 5⅜ x 8.
T143 Paperbound **$1.00**

NEW WORD PUZZLES, G. L. Kaufman. 100 ENTIRELY NEW puzzles based on words and their combinations that will delight crossword puzzle, Scrabble and Jotto fans. Chess words, based on the moves of the chess king; design-onyms, symmetrical designs made of synonyms; rhymed double-crostics; syllable sentences; addle letter anagrams; alphagrams; linkograms; and many others all brand new. Full solutions. Space to work problems. 196 figures. vi + 122pp. 5⅜ x 8.
T344 Paperbound **$1.00**

MAZES AND LABYRINTHS: A BOOK OF PUZZLES, W. Shepherd. Mazes, formerly associated with mystery and ritual, are still among the most intriguing of intellectual puzzles. This is a novel and different collection of 50 amusements that embody the principle of the maze: mazes in the classical tradition; 3-dimensional, ribbon, and Möbius-strip mazes; hidden messages; spatial arrangements; etc.—almost all built on amusing story situations. 84 illustrations. Essay on maze psychology. Solutions. xv + 122pp. 5⅜ x 8.
T731 Paperbound **$1.00**

MAGIC TRICKS & CARD TRICKS, W. Jonson. Two books bound as one. 52 tricks with cards, 37 tricks with coins, bills, eggs, smoke, ribbons, slates, etc. Details on presentation, misdirection, and routining will help you master such famous tricks as the Changing Card, Card in the Pocket, Four Aces, Coin Through the Hand, Bill in the Egg, Afghan Bands, and over 75 others. If you follow the lucid exposition and key diagrams carefully, you will finish these two books with an astonishing mastery of magic. 106 figures. 224pp. 5⅜ x 8. T909 Paperbound **$1.00**

PANORAMA OF MAGIC, Milbourne Christopher. A profusely illustrated history of stage magic, a unique selection of prints and engravings from the author's private collection of magic memorabilia, the largest of its kind. Apparatus, stage settings and costumes; ingenious ads distributed by the performers and satiric broadsides passed around in the streets ridiculing pompous showmen; programs; decorative souvenirs. The lively text, by one of America's foremost professional magicians, is full of anecdotes about almost legendary wizards: Dede, the Egyptian; Philadelphia, the wonder-worker; Robert-Houdin, "the father of modern magic;" Harry Houdini; scores more. Altogether a pleasure package for anyone interested in magic, stage setting and design, ethnology, psychology, or simply in unusual people. A Dover original. 295 illustrations; 8 in full color. Index. viii + 216pp. 8⅜ x 11¼.
T774 Paperbound **$2.25**

HOUDINI ON MAGIC, Harry Houdini. One of the greatest magicians of modern times explains his most prized secrets. How locks are picked, with illustrated picks and skeleton keys; how a girl is sawed into twins; how to walk through a brick wall — Houdini's explanations of 44 stage tricks with many diagrams. Also included is a fascinating discussion of great magicians of the past and the story of his fight against fraudulent mediums and spiritualists. Edited by W.B. Gibson and M.N. Young. Bibliography. 155 figures, photos. xv + 280pp. 5⅜ x 8.
T384 Paperbound **$1.35**

MATHEMATICS, MAGIC AND MYSTERY, Martin Gardner. Why do card tricks work? How do magicians perform astonishing mathematical feats? How is stage mind-reading possible? This is the first book length study explaining the application of probability, set theory, theory of numbers, topology, etc., to achieve many startling tricks. Non-technical, accurate, detailed! 115 sections discuss tricks with cards, dice, coins, knots, geometrical vanishing illusions, how a Curry square "demonstrates" that the sum of the parts may be greater than the whole, and dozens of others. No sleight of hand necessary! 135 illustrations. xii + 174pp. 5⅜ x 8.
T335 Paperbound **$1.00**

EASY-TO-DO ENTERTAINMENTS AND DIVERSIONS WITH COINS, CARDS, STRING, PAPER AND MATCHES, R. M. Abraham. Over 300 tricks, games and puzzles will provide young readers with absorbing fun. Sections on card games; paper-folding; tricks with coins, matches and pieces of string; games for the agile; toy-making from common household objects; mathematical recreations; and 50 miscellaneous pastimes. Anyone in charge of groups of youngsters, including hard-pressed parents, and in need of suggestions on how to keep children sensibly amused and quietly content will find this book indispensable. Clear, simple text, copious number of delightful line drawings and illustrative diagrams. Originally titled "Winter Nights Entertainments." Introduction by Lord Baden Powell. 329 illustrations. v + 186pp. 5⅜ x 8½.
T921 Paperbound **$1.00**

STRING FIGURES AND HOW TO MAKE THEM, Caroline Furness Jayne. 107 string figures plus variations selected from the best primitive and modern examples developed by Navajo, Apache, pygmies of Africa, Eskimo, in Europe, Australia, China, etc. The most readily understandable, easy-to-follow book in English on perennially popular recreation. Crystal-clear exposition; step-by-step diagrams. Everyone from kindergarten children to adults looking for unusual diversion will be endlessly amused. Index. Bibliography. Introduction by A. C. Haddon. 17 full-page plates. 960 illustrations. xxiii + 401pp. 5⅜ x 8½.
T152 Paperbound **$2.00**

Entertainments, Humor

ODDITIES AND CURIOSITIES OF WORDS AND LITERATURE, C. Bombaugh, edited by M. Gardner. The largest collection of idiosyncratic prose and poetry techniques in English, a legendary work in the curious and amusing bypaths of literary recreations and the play technique in literature—so important in modern works. Contains alphabetic poetry, acrostics, palindromes, scissors verse, centos, emblematic poetry, famous literary puns, hoaxes, notorious slips of the press, hilarious mistranslations, and much more. Revised and enlarged with modern material by Martin Gardner. 368pp. 5⅜ x 8. T759 Paperbound **$1.75**

A NONSENSE ANTHOLOGY, collected by Carolyn Wells. 245 of the best nonsense verses ever written, including nonsense puns, absurd arguments, mock epics and sagas, nonsense ballads, odes, "sick" verses, dog-Latin verses, French nonsense verses, songs. By Edward Lear, Lewis Carroll, Gelett Burgess, W. S. Gilbert, Hilaire Belloc, Peter Newell, Oliver Herford, etc., 83 writers in all plus over four score anonymous nonsense verses. A special section of limericks, plus famous nonsense such as Carroll's "Jabberwocky" and Lear's "The Jumblies" and much excellent verse virtually impossible to locate elsewhere. For 50 years considered the best anthology available. Index of first lines specially prepared for this edition. Introduction by Carolyn Wells. 3 indexes: Title, Author, First lines. xxxiii + 279pp. T499 Paperbound **$1.35**

THE BAD CHILD'S BOOK OF BEASTS, MORE BEASTS FOR WORSE CHILDREN, and A MORAL ALPHA-BET, H. Belloc. Hardly an anthology of humorous verse has appeared in the last 50 years without at least a couple of these famous nonsense verses. But one must see the entire volumes—with all the delightful original illustrations by Sir Basil Blackwood—to appreciate fully Belloc's charming and witty verses that play so subacidly on the platitudes of life and morals that beset his day—and ours. A great humor classic. Three books in one. Total of 157pp. 5⅜ x 8. T749 Paperbound **$1.00**

THE DEVIL'S DICTIONARY, Ambrose Bierce. Sardonic and irreverent barbs puncturing the pomposities and absurdities of American politics, business, religion, literature, and arts, by the country's greatest satirist in the classic tradition. Epigrammatic as Shaw, piercing as Swift, American as Mark Twain, Will Rogers, and Fred Allen, Bierce will always remain the favorite of a small coterie of enthusiasts, and of writers and speakers whom he supplies with "some of the most gorgeous witticisms of the English language" (H. L. Mencken). Over 1000 entries in alphabetical order. 144pp. 5⅜ x 8. T487 Paperbound **$1.00**

THE PURPLE COW AND OTHER NONSENSE, Gelett Burgess. The best of Burgess's early nonsense, selected from the first edition of the "Burgess Nonsense Book." Contains many of his most unusual and truly awe-inspiring pieces: 36 nonsense quatrains, the Poems of Patagonia, Alphabet of Famous Goops, and the other hilarious (and rare) adult nonsense that place him in the forefront of American humorists. All pieces are accompanied by the original Burgess illustrations. 123 illustrations. xiii + 113pp. 5⅜ x 8. T772 Paperbound **$1.00**

MY PIOUS FRIENDS AND DRUNKEN COMPANIONS and MORE PIOUS FRIENDS AND DRUNKEN COMPANIONS, Frank Shay. Folksingers, amateur and professional, and everyone who loves singing: here, available for the first time in 30 years, is this valued collection of 132 ballads, blues, vaudeville numbers, drinking songs, sea chanties, comedy songs. Songs of pre-Beatnik Bohemia; songs from all over America, England, France, Australia; the great songs of the Naughty Nineties and early twentieth-century America. Over a third with music. Woodcuts by John Held, Jr. convey perfectly the brash insouciance of an era of rollicking unabashed song. 12 illustrations by John Held, Jr. Two indexes (Titles and First lines and Choruses). Introductions by the author. Two volumes bound as one. Total of xvi + 235pp. 5⅜ x 8½. T946 Paperbound **$1.25**

HOW TO TELL THE BIRDS FROM THE FLOWERS, R. W. Wood. How not to confuse a carrot with a parrot, a grape with an ape, a puffin with nuffin. Delightful drawings, clever puns, absurd little poems point out far-fetched resemblances in nature. The author was a leading physicist. Introduction by Margaret Wood White. 106 illus. 60pp. 5⅜ x 8. T523 Paperbound **75¢**

PECK'S BAD BOY AND HIS PA, George W. Peck. The complete edition, containing both volumes, of one of the most widely read American humor books. The endless ingenious pranks played by bad boy "Hennery" on his pa and the grocery man, the outraged pomposity of Pa, the perpetual ridiculing of middle class institutions, are as entertaining today as they were in 1883. No pale sophistications or subtleties, but rather humor vigorous, raw, earthy, imaginative, and, as folk humor often is, sadistic. This peculiarly fascinating book is also valuable to historians and students of American culture as a portrait of an age. 100 original illustrations by True Williams. Introduction by E. F. Bleiler. 347pp. 5⅜ x 8. T497 Paperbound **$1.50**

THE HUMOROUS VERSE OF LEWIS CARROLL. Almost every poem Carroll ever wrote, the largest collection ever published, including much never published elsewhere: 150 parodies, burlesques, riddles, ballads, acrostics, etc., with 130 original illustrations by Tenniel, Carroll, and others. "Addicts will be grateful . . . there is nothing for the faithful to do but sit down and fall to the banquet," N. Y. Times. Index to first lines. xiv + 446pp. 5⅜ x 8.
T654 Paperbound **$2.00**

DIVERSIONS AND DIGRESSIONS OF LEWIS CARROLL. A major new treasure for Carroll fans! Rare privately published humor, fantasy, puzzles, and games by Carroll at his whimsical best, with a new vein of frank satire. Includes many new mathematical amusements and recreations, among them the fragmentary Part III of "Curiosa Mathematica." Contains "The Rectory Umbrella," "The New Belfry," "The Vision of the Three T's," and much more. New 32-page supplement of rare photographs taken by Carroll. x + 375pp. 5⅜ x 8.
T732 Paperbound **$2.00**

THE COMPLETE NONSENSE OF EDWARD LEAR. This is the only complete edition of this master of gentle madness available at a popular price. A BOOK OF NONSENSE, NONSENSE SONGS, MORE NONSENSE SONGS AND STORIES in their entirety with all the old favorites that have delighted children and adults for years. The Dong With A Luminous Nose, The Jumblies, The Owl and the Pussycat, and hundreds of other bits of wonderful nonsense. 214 limericks, 3 sets of Nonsense Botany, 5 Nonsense Alphabets, 546 drawings by Lear himself, and much more. 320pp. 5⅜ x 8.
T167 Paperbound **$1.00**

THE MELANCHOLY LUTE, The Humorous Verse of Franklin P. Adams ("FPA"). The author's own selection of light verse, drawn from thirty years of FPA's column, "The Conning Tower," syndicated all over the English-speaking world. Witty, perceptive, literate, these ninety-six poems range from parodies of other poets, Millay, Longfellow, Edgar Guest, Kipling, Masefield, etc., and free and hilarious translations of Horace and other Latin poets, to satiric comments on fabled American institutions—the New York Subways, preposterous ads, suburbanites, sensational journalism, etc. They reveal with vigor and clarity the humor, integrity and restraint of a wise and gentle American satirist. Introduction by Robert Hutchinson. vi + 122pp. 5⅜ x 8½.
T108 Paperbound **$1.00**

SINGULAR TRAVELS, CAMPAIGNS, AND ADVENTURES OF BARON MUNCHAUSEN, R. E. Raspe, with 90 illustrations by Gustave Doré. The first edition in over 150 years to reestablish the deeds of the Prince of Liars exactly as Raspe first recorded them in 1785—the genuine Baron Munchausen, one of the most popular personalities in English literature. Included also are the best of the many sequels, written by other hands. Introduction on Raspe by J. Carswell. Bibliography of early editions. xliv + 192pp. 5⅜ x 8.
T698 Paperbound **$1.00**

THE WIT AND HUMOR OF OSCAR WILDE, ed. by Alvin Redman. Wilde at his most brilliant, in 1000 epigrams exposing weaknesses and hypocrisies of "civilized" society. Divided into 49 categories—sin, wealth, women, America, etc.—to aid writers, speakers. Includes excerpts from his trials, books, plays, criticism. Formerly "The Epigrams of Oscar Wilde." Introduction by Vyvyan Holland, Wilde's only living son. Introductory essay by editor. 260pp. 5⅜ x 8.
T602 Paperbound **$1.00**

MAX AND MORITZ, Wilhelm Busch. Busch is one of the great humorists of all time, as well as the father of the modern comic strip. This volume, translated by H. A. Klein and other hands, contains the perennial favorite "Max and Moritz" (translated by C. T. Brooks), Plisch and Plum, Das Rabennest, Eispeter, and seven other whimsical, sardonic, jovial, diabolical cartoon and verse stories. Lively English translations parallel the original German. This work has delighted millions since it first appeared in the 19th century, and is guaranteed to please almost anyone. Edited by H. A. Klein, with an afterword. x + 205pp. 5⅝ x 8½.
T181 Paperbound **$1.15**

HYPOCRITICAL HELENA, Wilhelm Busch. A companion volume to "Max and Moritz," with the title piece (Die Fromme Helena) and 10 other highly amusing cartoon and verse stories, all newly translated by H. A. Klein and M. C. Klein: Adventure on New Year's Eve (Abenteuer in der Neujahrsnacht), Hangover on the Morning after New Year's Eve (Der Katzenjammer am Neujahrsmorgen), etc. English and German in parallel columns. Hours of pleasure, also a fine language aid. x + 205pp. 5⅝ x 8½.
T184 Paperbound **$1.00**

THE BEAR THAT WASN'T, Frank Tashlin. What does it mean? Is it simply delightful wry humor, or a charming story of a bear who wakes up in the midst of a factory, or a satire on Big Business, or an existential cartoon-story of the human condition, or a symbolization of the struggle between conformity and the individual? New York Herald Tribune said of the first edition: ". . . a fable for grownups that will be fun for children. Sit down with the book and get your own bearings." Long an underground favorite with readers of all ages and opinions. v + 51pp. Illustrated. 5⅜ x 8½.
T939 Paperbound **75¢**

RUTHLESS RHYMES FOR HEARTLESS HOMES and MORE RUTHLESS RHYMES FOR HEARTLESS HOMES, Harry Graham ("Col. D. Streamer"). Two volumes of Little Willy and 48 other poetic disasters. A bright, new reprint of oft-quoted, never forgotten, devastating humor by a precursor of today's "sick" joke school. For connoisseurs of wicked, wacky humor and all who delight in the comedy of manners. Original drawings are a perfect complement. 61 illustrations. Index. vi + 69pp. Two vols. bound as one. 5⅜ x 8½.
T930 Paperbound **75¢**

Say It language phrase books

These handy phrase books (128 to 196 pages each) make grammatical drills unnecessary for an elementary knowledge of a spoken foreign language. Covering most matters of travel and everyday life each volume contains:

Over 1000 phrases and sentences in immediately useful forms — foreign language plus English.

Modern usage designed for Americans. Specific phrases like, "Give me small change," and "Please call a taxi."

Simplified phonetic transcription you will be able to read at sight.

The only completely indexed phrase books on the market.

Covers scores of important situations: — Greetings, restaurants, sightseeing, useful expressions, etc.

These books are prepared by native linguists who are professors at Columbia, N.Y.U., Fordham and other great universities. Use them independently or with any other book or record course. They provide a supplementary living element that most other courses lack. Individual volumes in:

Russian 75¢	Italian 75¢	Spanish 75¢	German 75¢
Hebrew 75¢	Danish 75¢	Japanese 75¢	Swedish 75¢
Dutch 75¢	Esperanto 75¢	Modern Greek 75¢	Portuguese 75¢
Norwegian 75¢	Polish 75¢	French 75¢	Yiddish 75¢
Turkish 75¢		English for German-speaking people 75¢	
English for Italian-speaking people 75¢		English for Spanish-speaking people 75¢	

Large clear type. 128-196 pages each. 3½ x 5¼. Sturdy paper binding.

Listen and Learn language records

LISTEN & LEARN is the only language record course designed especially to meet your travel and everyday needs. It is available in separate sets for FRENCH, SPANISH, GERMAN, JAPANESE, RUSSIAN, MODERN GREEK, PORTUGUESE, ITALIAN and HEBREW, and each set contains three 33⅓ rpm long-playing records—1½ hours of recorded speech by eminent native speakers who are professors at Columbia, New York University, Queens College.

Check the following special features found only in LISTEN & LEARN:

- **Dual-language recording. 812 selected phrases and sentences**, over 3200 words, spoken first in English, then in their foreign language equivalents. A suitable pause follows each foreign phrase, allowing you time to repeat the expression. You learn by unconscious assimilation.
- **128 to 206-page manual** contains everything on the records, plus a simple phonetic pronunciation guide.
- **Indexed for convenience. The only set on the market** that is completely indexed. No more puzzling over where to find the phrase you need. Just look in the rear of the manual.
- **Practical.** No time wasted on material you can find in any grammar. LISTEN & LEARN covers central core material with phrase approach. Ideal for the person with limited learning time.
- **Living, modern expressions**, not found in other courses. Hygienic products, modern equipment, shopping—expressions used every day, like "nylon" and "air-conditioned."
- **Limited objective.** Everything you learn, no matter where you stop, is immediately useful. You have to finish other courses, wade through grammar and vocabulary drill, before they help you.
- **High-fidelity recording.** LISTEN & LEARN records equal in clarity and surface-silence any record on the market costing up to $6.

"Excellent . . . the spoken records . . . impress me as being among the very best on the market," **Prof. Mario Pei**, Dept. of Romance Languages, Columbia University. "Inexpensive and well-done . . . it would make an ideal present," CHICAGO SUNDAY TRIBUNE. "More genuinely helpful than anything of its kind which I have previously encountered," **Sidney Clark**, well-known author of "ALL THE BEST" travel books.

UNCONDITIONAL GUARANTEE. Try LISTEN & LEARN, then return it within 10 days for full refund if you are not satisfied.

Each set contains three twelve-inch 33⅓ records, manual, and album.

SPANISH	the set $5.95	GERMAN	the set $5.95
FRENCH	the set $5.95	ITALIAN	the set $5.95
RUSSIAN	the set $5.95	JAPANESE	the set $6.95
PORTUGUESE	the set $5.95	MODERN GREEK	the set $5.95
MODERN HEBREW	the set $5.95		

Americana

THE EYES OF DISCOVERY, J. Bakeless. A vivid reconstruction of how unspoiled America appeared to the first white men. Authentic and enlightening accounts of Hudson's landing in New York, Coronado's trek through the Southwest; scores of explorers, settlers, trappers, soldiers. America's pristine flora, fauna, and Indians in every region and state in fresh and unusual new aspects. "A fascinating view of what the land was like before the first highway went through," Time. 68 contemporary illustrations, 39 newly added in this edition. Index. Bibliography. x + 500pp. 5⅜ x 8.   T761 Paperbound $2.25

AUDUBON AND HIS JOURNALS, J. J. Audubon. A collection of fascinating accounts of Europe and America in the early 1800's through Audubon's own eyes. Includes the Missouri River Journals —an eventful trip through America's untouched heartland, the Labrador Journals, the European Journals, the famous "Episodes", and other rare Audubon material, including the descriptive chapters from the original letterpress edition of the "Ornithological Studies", omitted in all later editions. Indispensable for ornithologists, naturalists, and all lovers of Americana and adventure. 70-page biography by Audubon's granddaughter. 38 illustrations. Index. Total of 1106pp. 5⅜ x 8.   T675 Vol I Paperbound $2.25
T676 Vol II Paperbound $2.25
The set $4.50

TRAVELS OF WILLIAM BARTRAM, edited by Mark Van Doren. The first inexpensive illustrated edition of one of the 18th century's most delightful books is an excellent source of first-hand material on American geography, anthropology, and natural history. Many descriptions of early Indian tribes are our only source of information on them prior to the infiltration of the white man. "The mind of a scientist with the soul of a poet," John Livingston Lowes. 13 original illustrations and maps. Edited with an introduction by Mark Van Doren. 448pp. 5⅜ x 8.
T13 Paperbound $2.00

GARRETS AND PRETENDERS: A HISTORY OF BOHEMIANISM IN AMERICA, A. Parry. The colorful and fantastic history of American Bohemianism from Poe to Kerouac. This is the only complete record of hoboes, cranks, starving poets, and suicides. Here are Pfaff, Whitman, Crane, Bierce, Pound, and many others. New chapters by the author and by H. T. Moore bring this thorough and well-documented history down to the Beatniks. "An excellent account," N. Y. Times. Scores of cartoons, drawings, and caricatures. Bibliography. Index. xxviii + 421pp. 5⅝ x 8⅜.   T708 Paperbound $1.95

THE EXPLORATION OF THE COLORADO RIVER AND ITS CANYONS, J. W. Powell. The thrilling first-hand account of the expedition that filled in the last white space on the map of the United States. Rapids, famine, hostile Indians, and mutiny are among the perils encountered as the unknown Colorado Valley reveals its secrets. This is the only uncut version of Major Powell's classic of exploration that has been printed in the last 60 years. Includes later reflections and subsequent expedition. 250 illustrations, new map. 400pp. 5⅝ x 8⅜.
T94 Paperbound $2.25

THE JOURNAL OF HENRY D. THOREAU, Edited by Bradford Torrey and Francis H. Allen. Henry Thoreau is not only one of the most important figures in American literature and social thought; his voluminous journals (from which his books emerged as selections and crystallizations) constitute both the longest, most sensitive record of personal internal development and a most penetrating description of a historical moment in American culture. This present set, which was first issued in fourteen volumes, contains Thoreau's entire journals from 1837 to 1862, with the exception of the lost years which were found only recently. We are reissuing it, complete and unabridged, with a new introduction by Walter Harding, Secretary of the Thoreau Society. Fourteen volumes reissued in two volumes. Foreword by Henry Seidel Canby. Total of 1888pp. 8⅜ x 12¼.   T312-3 Two volume set, Clothbound $20.00

GAMES AND SONGS OF AMERICAN CHILDREN, collected by William Wells Newell. A remarkable collection of 190 games with songs that accompany many of them; cross references to show similarities, differences among them; variations; musical notation for 38 songs. Textual discussions show relations with folk-drama and other aspects of folk tradition. Grouped into categories for ready comparative study: Love-games, histories, playing at work, human life, bird and beast, mythology, guessing-games, etc. New introduction covers relations of songs and dances to timeless heritage of folklore, biographical sketch of Newell, other pertinent data. A good source of inspiration for those in charge of groups of children and a valuable reference for anthropologists, sociologists, psychiatrists. Introduction by Carl Withers. New indexes of first lines, games. 5⅜ x 8½. xii + 242pp.   T354 Paperbound $1.75

Art, History of Art, Antiques,
Graphic Arts, Handcrafts

ART STUDENTS' ANATOMY, E. J. Farris. Outstanding art anatomy that uses chiefly living objects for its illustrations. 71 photos of undraped men, women, children are accompanied by carefully labeled matching sketches to illustrate the skeletal system, articulations and movements, bony landmarks, the muscular system, skin, fasciae, fat, etc. 9 x-ray photos show movement of joints. Undraped models are shown in such actions as serving in tennis, drawing a bow in archery, playing football, dancing, preparing to spring and to dive. Also discussed and illustrated are proportions, age and sex differences, the anatomy of the smile, etc. 8 plates by the great early 18th century anatomic illustrator Siegfried Albinus are also included. Glossary. 158 figures, 7 in color. x + 159pp. 5⅝ x 8⅜.   T744 Paperbound **$1.50**

AN ATLAS OF ANATOMY FOR ARTISTS, F Schider. A new 3rd edition of this standard text enlarged by 52 new illustrations of hands, anatomical studies by Cloquet, and expressive life studies of the body by Barcsay. 189 clear, detailed plates offer you precise information of impeccable accuracy. 29 plates show all aspects of the skeleton, with closeups of special areas, while 54 full-page plates, mostly in two colors, give human musculature as seen from four different points of view, with cutaways for important portions of the body. 14 full-page plates provide photographs of hand forms, eyelids, female breasts, and indicate the location of muscles upon models. 59 additional plates show how great artists of the past utilized human anatomy. They reproduce sketches and finished work by such artists as Michelangelo, Leonardo da Vinci, Goya, and 15 others. This is a lifetime reference work which will be one of the most important books in any artist's library. "The standard reference tool," AMERICAN LIBRARY ASSOCIATION. "Excellent," AMERICAN ARTIST. Third enlarged edition. 189 plates, 647 illustrations. xxvi + 192pp. 7⅞ x 10⅝.   T241 Clothbound **$6.00**

AN ATLAS OF ANIMAL ANATOMY FOR ARTISTS, W. Ellenberger, H. Baum, H. Dittrich. The largest, richest animal anatomy for artists available in English. 99 detailed anatomical plates of such animals as the horse, dog, cat, lion, deer, seal, kangaroo, flying squirrel, cow, bull, goat, monkey, hare, and bat. Surface features are clearly indicated, while progressive beneath-the-skin pictures show musculature, tendons, and bone structure. Rest and action are exhibited in terms of musculature and skeletal structure and detailed cross-sections are given for heads and important features. The animals chosen are representative of specific families so that a study of these anatomies will provide knowledge of hundreds of related species. "Highly recommended as one of the very few books on the subject worthy of being used as an authoritative guide," DESIGN. "Gives a fundamental knowledge," AMERICAN ARTIST. Second revised, enlarged edition with new plates from Cuvier, Stubbs, etc. 288 illustrations. 153pp. 11⅜ x 9.   T82 Clothbound **$6.00**

THE HUMAN FIGURE IN MOTION, Eadweard Muybridge. The largest selection in print of Muybridge's famous high-speed action photos of the human figure in motion. 4789 photographs illustrate 162 different actions: men, women, children—mostly undraped—are shown walking, running, carrying various objects, sitting, lying down, climbing, throwing, arising, and performing over 100 other actions. Some actions are shown in as many as 150 photographs each. All in all there are more than 500 action strips in this enormous volume, series shots taken at shutter speeds of as high as 1/6000th of a second! These are not posed shots, but true stopped motion. They show bone and muscle in situations that the human eye is not fast enough to capture. Earlier, smaller editions of these prints have brought $40 and more on the out-of-print market. "A must for artists," ART IN FOCUS. "An unparalleled dictionary of action for all artists," AMERICAN ARTIST. 390 full-page plates, with 4789 photographs. Printed on heavy glossy stock. Reinforced binding with headbands. xxi + 390pp. 7⅞ x 10⅝.   T204 Clothbound **$10.00**

ANIMALS IN MOTION, Eadweard Muybridge. This is the largest collection of animal action photos in print. 34 different animals (horses, mules, oxen, goats, camels, pigs, cats, guanacos, lions, gnus, deer, monkeys, eagles—and 21 others) in 132 characteristic actions. The horse alone is shown in more than 40 different actions. All 3919 photographs are taken in series at speeds up to 1/6000th of a second. The secrets of leg motion, spinal patterns, head movements, strains and contortions shown nowhere else are captured. You will see exactly how a lion sets his foot down; how an elephant's knees are a human's—and how they differ; the position of a kangaroo's legs in mid-leap; how an ostrich's head bobs; details of the flight of birds—and thousands of facets of motion only the fastest cameras can catch. Photographed from domestic animals and animals in the Philadelphia zoo, it contains neither semiposed artificial shots nor distorted telephoto shots taken under adverse conditions. Artists, biologists, decorators, cartoonists, will find this book indispensable for understanding animals in motion. "A really marvelous series of plates," NATURE (London). "The dry plate's most spectacular early use was by Eadweard Muybridge," LIFE. 3919 photographs; 380 full pages of plates. 440pp. Printed on heavy glossy paper. Deluxe binding with headbands. 7⅞ x 10⅝.   T203 Clothbound **$10.00**

THE AUTOBIOGRAPHY OF AN IDEA, Louis Sullivan. The pioneer architect whom Frank Lloyd Wright called "the master" reveals an acute sensitivity to social forces and values in this passionately honest account. He records the crystallization of his opinions and theories, the growth of his organic theory of architecture that still influences American designers and architects, contemporary ideas, etc. This volume contains the first appearance of 34 full-page plates of his finest architecture. Unabridged reissue of 1924 edition. New introduction by R. M. Line. Index. xiv + 335pp. 5⅜ x 8. T281 Paperbound **$2.00**

THE DRAWINGS OF HEINRICH KLEY. The first uncut republication of both of Kley's devastating sketchbooks, which first appeared in pre-World War I Germany. One of the greatest cartoonists and social satirists of modern times, his exuberant and iconoclastic fantasy and his extra-ordinary technique place him in the great tradition of Bosch, Breughel, and Goya, while his subject matter has all the immediacy and tension of our century. 200 drawings. viii + 128pp. 7¾ x 10¾. T24 Paperbound **$1.85**

MORE DRAWINGS BY HEINRICH KLEY. All the sketches from Leut' Und Viecher (1912) and Sammel-Album (1923) not included in the previous Dover edition of Drawings. More of the bizarre, mercilessly iconoclastic sketches that shocked and amused on their original publica-tion. Nothing was too sacred, no one too eminent for satirization by this imaginative, in-dividual and accomplished master cartoonist. A total of 158 illustrations. Iv + 104pp. 7¾ x 10¾. T41 Paperbound **$1.85**

PINE FURNITURE OF EARLY NEW ENGLAND, R. H. Kettell. A rich understanding of one of America's most original folk arts that collectors of antiques, interior decorators, craftsmen, woodworkers, and everyone interested in American history and art will find fascinating and immensely useful. 413 illustrations of more than 300 chairs, benches, racks, beds, cupboards, mirrors, shelves, tables, and other furniture will show all the simple beauty and character of early New England furniture. 55 detailed drawings carefully analyze outstanding pieces. "With its rich store of illustrations, this book emphasizes the individuality and varied design of early American pine furniture. It should be welcomed," ANTIQUES. 413 illustrations and 55 working drawings. 475. 8 x 10¾. T145 Clothbound **$10.00**

THE HUMAN FIGURE, J. H. Vanderpoel. Every important artistic element of the human figure is pointed out in minutely detailed word descriptions in this classic text and illustrated as well in 430 pencil and charcoal drawings. Thus the text of this book directs your attention to all the characteristic features and subtle differences of the male and female (adults, children, and aged persons), as though a master artist were telling you what to look for at each stage. 2nd edition, revised and enlarged by George Bridgman. Foreword. 430 illustrations. 143pp. 6⅛ x 9¼. T432 Paperbound **$1.50**

LETTERING AND ALPHABETS, J. A. Cavanagh. This unabridged reissue of LETTERING offers a full discussion, analysis, illustration of 89 basic hand lettering styles — styles derived from Caslons, Bodonis, Garamonds, Gothic, Black Letter, Oriental, and many others. Upper and lower cases, numerals and common signs pictured. Hundreds of technical hints on make-up, construction, artistic validity, strokes, pens, brushes, white areas, etc. May be reproduced without permission! 89 complete alphabets; 72 lettered specimens. 121pp. 9⅜ x 8. T53 Paperbound **$1.35**

STICKS AND STONES, Lewis Mumford. A survey of the forces that have conditioned American architecture and altered its forms. The author discusses the medieval tradition in early New England villages; the Renaissance influence which developed with the rise of the merchant class; the classical influence of Jefferson's time; the "Mechanicsvilles" of Poe's generation; the Brown Decades; the philosophy of the Imperial facade; and finally the modern machine age. "A truly remarkable book," SAT. REV. OF LITERATURE. 2nd revised edition. 21 illustra-tions. xvii + 228pp. 5⅜ x 8. T202 Paperbound **$1.75**

THE STANDARD BOOK OF QUILT MAKING AND COLLECTING, Marguerite Ickis. A complete easy-to-follow guide with all the information you need to make beautiful, useful quilts. How to plan, design, cut, sew, appliqué, avoid sewing problems, use rag bag, make borders, tuft, every other aspect. Over 100 traditional quilts shown, including over 40 full-size patterns. At-home hobby for fun, profit. Index. 483 illus. 1 color plate. 287pp. 6¾ x 9½. T582 Paperbound **$2.00**

THE BOOK OF SIGNS, Rudolf Koch. Formerly $20 to $25 on the out-of-print market, now only $1.00 in this unabridged new edition! 493 symbols from ancient manuscripts, medieval cathe-drals, coins, catacombs, pottery, etc. Crosses, monograms of Roman emperors, astrological, chemical, botanical, runes, housemarks, and 7 other categories. Invaluable for handicraft workers, illustrators, scholars, etc., this material may be reproduced without permission. 493 illustrations by Fritz Kredel. 104pp. 6½ x 9¼. T162 Paperbound **$1.00**

PRIMITIVE ART, Franz Boas. This authoritative and exhaustive work by a great American anthropologist covers the entire gamut of primitive art. Pottery, leatherwork, metal work, stone work, wood, basketry, are treated in detail. Theories of primitive art, historical depth in art history, technical virtuosity, unconscious levels of patterning, symbolism, styles, litera-ture, music, dance, etc. A must book for the interested layman, the anthropologist, artist, handicrafter (hundreds of unusual motifs), and the historian. Over 900 illustrations (50 ceramic vessels, 12 totem poles, etc.). 376pp. 5⅜ x 8. T25 Paperbound **$2.25**

Fiction

FLATLAND, E. A. Abbott. A science-fiction classic of life in a 2-dimensional world that is also a first-rate introduction to such aspects of modern science as relativity and hyperspace. Political, moral, satirical, and humorous overtones have made FLATLAND fascinating reading for thousands. 7th edition. New introduction by Banesh Hoffmann. 16 illustrations. 128pp. 5⅜ x 8.   T1 Paperbound **$1.00**

THE WONDERFUL WIZARD OF OZ, L. F. Baum. Only edition in print with all the original W. W. Denslow illustrations in full color—as much a part of "The Wizard" as Tenniel's drawings are of "Alice in Wonderland." "The Wizard" is still America's best-loved fairy tale, in which, as the author expresses it, "The wonderment and joy are retained and the heartaches and night-mares left out." Now today's young readers can enjoy every word and wonderful picture of the original book. New introduction by Martin Gardner. A Baum bibliography. 23 full-page color plates. viii + 268pp. 5⅜ x 8.   T691 Paperbound **$1.50**

THE MARVELOUS LAND OF OZ, L. F. Baum. This is the equally enchanting sequel to the "Wizard," continuing the adventures of the Scarecrow and the Tin Woodman. The hero this time is a little boy named Tip, and all the delightful Oz magic is still present. This is the Oz book with the Animated Saw-Horse, the Woggle-Bug, and Jack Pumpkinhead. All the original John R. Neill illustrations, 10 in full color. 287 pp. 5⅜ x 8.   T692 Paperbound **$1.50**

28 SCIENCE FICTION STORIES OF H. G. WELLS. Two full unabridged novels, MEN LIKE GODS and STAR BEGOTTEN, plus 26 short stories by the master science-fiction writer of all time! Stories of space, time, invention, exploration, future adventure—an indispensable part of the library of everyone interested in science and adventure. PARTIAL CONTENTS: Men Like Gods, The Country of the Blind, In the Abyss, The Crystal Egg, The Man Who Could Work Miracles, A Story of the Days to Come, The Valley of Spiders, and 21 more! 928pp. 5⅜ x 8.
T265 Clothbound **$4.50**

THREE MARTIAN NOVELS, Edgar Rice Burroughs. Contains: Thuvia, Maid of Mars; The Chessmen of Mars; and The Master Mind of Mars. High adventure set in an imaginative and intricate conception of the Red Planet. Mars is peopled with an intelligent, heroic human race which lives in densely populated cities and with fierce barbarians who inhabit dead sea bottoms. Other exciting creatures abound amidst an inventive framework of Martian history and geography. Complete unabridged reprintings of the first edition. 16 illustrations by J. Allen St. John. vi + 499pp. 5⅜ x 8½.   T39 Paperbound **$1.85**

SEVEN SCIENCE FICTION NOVELS, H. G. Wells. Full unabridged texts of 7 science-fiction novels of the master. Ranging from biology, physics, chemistry, astronomy to sociology and other studies, Mr. Wells extrapolates whole worlds of strange and intriguing character. "One will have to go far to match this for entertainment, excitement, and sheer pleasure . . . ," NEW YORK TIMES. Contents: The Time Machine, The Island of Dr. Moreau, First Men in the Moon, The Invisible Man, The War of the Worlds, The Food of the Gods, In the Days of the Comet. 1015pp. 5⅜ x 8.   T264 Clothbound **$4.50**

THE LAND THAT TIME FORGOT and THE MOON MAID, Edgar Rice Burroughs. In the opinion of many, Burroughs' best work. The first concerns a strange island where evolution is individual rather than phylogenetic. Speechless anthropoids develop into intelligent human beings within a single generation. The second projects the reader far into the future and describes the first voyage to the Moon (in the year 2025), the conquest of the Earth by the Moon, and years of violence and adventure as the enslaved Earthmen try to regain possession of their planet. "An imaginative tour de force that keeps the reader keyed up and expectant," NEW YORK TIMES. Complete, unabridged text of the original two novels (three parts in each). 5 illustrations by J. Allen St. John. vi + 552pp. 5⅜ x 8½.
T1020 Clothbound **$3.75**
T358 Paperbound **$2.00**

3 ADVENTURE NOVELS by H. Rider Haggard. Complete texts of "She," "King Solomon's Mines," "Allan Quatermain." Qualities of discovery; desire for immortality; search for primitive, for what is unadorned by civilization, have kept these novels of African adventure exciting, alive to readers from R. L. Stevenson to George Orwell. 636pp. 5⅜ x 8.
T584 Paperbound **$2.00**

A PRINCESS OF MARS and A FIGHTING MAN OF MARS: TWO MARTIAN NOVELS BY EDGAR RICE BURROUGHS. "Princess of Mars" is the very first of the great Martian novels written by Burroughs, and it is probably the best of them all; it set the pattern for all of his later fantasy novels and contains a thrilling cast of strange peoples and creatures and the formula of Olympian heroism amidst ever-fluctuating fortunes which Burroughs carries off so successfully. "Fighting Man" returns to the same scenes and cities—many years later. A mad scientist, a degenerate dictator, and an indomitable defender of the right clash—with the fate of the Red Planet at stake! Complete, unabridged reprinting of original editions. Illustrations by F. E. Schoonover and Hugh Hutton. v + 356pp. 5⅜ x 8½.
T1140 Paperbound **$1.75**

Music

A GENERAL HISTORY OF MUSIC, Charles Burney. A detailed coverage of music from the Greeks up to 1789, with full information on all types of music: sacred and secular, vocal and instrumental, operatic and symphonic. Theory, notation, forms, instruments, innovators, composers, performers, typical and important works, and much more in an easy, entertaining style. Burney covered much of Europe and spoke with hundreds of authorities and composers so that this work is more than a compilation of records . . . it is a living work of careful and first-hand scholarship. Its account of thoroughbass (18th century) Italian music is probably still the best introduction on the subject. A recent NEW YORK TIMES review said, "Surprisingly few of Burney's statements have been invalidated by modern research . . . still of great value." Edited and corrected by Frank Mercer. 35 figures. Indices. 1915pp. 5⅜ x 8. 2 volumes. T36 The Set, Clothbound **$12.50**

A DICTIONARY OF HYMNOLOGY, John Julian. This exhaustive and scholarly work has become known as an invaluable source of hundreds of thousands of important and often difficult to obtain facts on the history and use of hymns in the western world. Everyone interested in hymns will be fascinated by the accounts of famous hymns and hymn writers and amazed by the amount of practical information he will find. More than 30,000 entries on individual hymns, giving authorship, date and circumstances of composition, publication, textual variations, translations, denominational and ritual usage, etc. Biographies of more than 9,000 hymn writers, and essays on important topics such as Christmas carols and children's hymns, and much other unusual and valuable information. A 200 page double-columned index of first lines — the largest in print. Total of 1786 pages in two reinforced clothbound volumes. 6¼ x 9¼. The set, T333 Clothbound **$17.50**

MUSIC IN MEDIEVAL BRITAIN, F. Ll. Harrison. The most thorough, up-to-date, and accurate treatment of the subject ever published, beautifully illustrated. Complete account of institutions and choirs; carols, masses, and motets; liturgy and plainsong; and polyphonic music from the Norman Conquest to the Reformation. Discusses the various schools of music and their reciprocal influences; the origin and development of new ritual forms; development and use of instruments; and new evidence on many problems of the period. Reproductions of scores, over 200 excerpts from medieval melodies. Rules of harmony and dissonance; influence of Continental styles; great composers (Dunstable, Cornysh, Fairfax, etc.); and much more. Register and index of more than 400 musicians. Index of titles. General Index. 225-item bibliography. 6 Appendices. xix + 491pp. 5⅝ x 8¾. T705 Clothbound **$10.00**

THE MUSIC OF SPAIN, Gilbert Chase. Only book in English to give concise, comprehensive account of Iberian music; new Chapter covers music since 1941. Victoria, Albéniz, Cabezón, Pedrell, Turina, hundreds of other composers; popular and folk music; the Gypsies; the guitar; dance, theatre, opera, with only extensive discussion in English of the Zarzuela; virtuosi such as Casals; much more. "Distinguished . . . readable," Saturday Review. 400-item bibliography. Index. 27 photos. 383pp. 5⅜ x 8. T549 Paperbound **$2.25**

ON STUDYING SINGING, Sergius Kagen. An intelligent method of voice-training, which leads you around pitfalls that waste your time, money, and effort. Exposes rigid, mechanical systems, baseless theories, deleterious exercises. "Logical, clear, convincing . . . dead right," Virgil Thomson, N.Y. Herald Tribune. "I recommend this volume highly," Maggie Teyte, Saturday Review. 119pp. 5⅜ x 8. T622 Paperbound **$1.35**

Prices subject to change without notice.

Dover publishes books on art, music, philosophy, literature, languages, history, social sciences, psychology, handcrafts, orientalia, puzzles and entertainments, chess, pets and gardens, books explaining science, intermediate and higher mathematics, mathematical physics, engineering, biological sciences, earth sciences, classics of science, etc. Write to:

Dept. catrr.
Dover Publications, Inc.
180 Varick Street, N.Y. 14, N.Y.